KU-756-908

Royal Society of Medicine

*International Congress and Symposium Series*

*Number 76*

# Benign breast disease

*Edited by*

## M. BAUM
## W. D. GEORGE
## L. E. HUGHES

1984

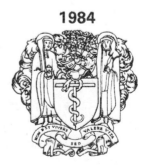

*Published by*

**THE ROYAL SOCIETY OF MEDICINE**
1 Wimpole Street, London

ROYAL SOCIETY OF MEDICINE
1 Wimpole Street, London W1M 8AE


Distributed by
OXFORD UNIVERSITY PRESS
Walton Street, Oxford OX2 6DP
London New York Toronto
Delhi Bombay Calcutta Madras Karachi
Kuala Lumpur Singapore Hong Kong Tokyo
Nairobi Dar es Salaam Cape Town
Melbourne Auckland

and associated companies in
Beirut Berlin Ibadan Mexico City Nicosia

Oxford is a trade mark of Oxford University Press

Copyright © 1983 by

ROYAL SOCIETY OF MEDICINE

British Library Cataloguing in Publication Data
Benign breast disease.—(Royal Society of Medicine
    international congress and symposium series; no. 76)
    1. Breast—Diseases
    I. Baum, Michael   II. George, W. D.
    III. Hughes, L. E.   IV. Winthrop Laboratories
    V. Series
    618.1'9     RG491
    ISBN 0–19–922036–0

Printed in Great Britain by Latimer Trend and Co. Ltd, Plymouth

**Royal Society of Medicine**

*International Congress and Symposium Series*
Editor-in-Chief: H. J. C. J. L'Etang

*Number 76*

# Benign breast disease

---

*Proceedings of an International Symposium
sponsored by Winthrop Laboratories held in Florence,
Italy, on 25–26 March 1983.*

# Contributors

*SYMPOSIUM CHAIRMAN*

The Rt. Hon. The Lord Porritt GCMG, GCVO, CBE

*CHAIRMEN OF SESSIONS*

**Professor M. Baum**
> King's College Hospital Medical School, London, England

**Professor W. D. George**
> University of Glasgow and Western Infirmary, Glasgow, Scotland

**Professor L. E. Hughes**
> Welsh National School of Medicine, University Department of Surgery, Cardiff, Wales

*SPEAKERS*

**Dr A. Audebert**
> Institut Aquitain de Recherche et d'etude en Reproduction Humaine, 40 Cour de Verdun, Bordeaux, France

**Professor M. Baum**
> Professor Surgery, King's College, Hospital Medical School, Denmark Hill, London SE5 8RX

**Mr E. A. Benson FRCS**
> The General Infirmary at Leeds, Great George Street, Leeds 1, West Yorkshire

**Dr A. Doberl**
> Department of Clinical Research, Sterling Winthrop, Scandinavia, Solna, Sweden

**Dr H. Duguid**
> Dundee Royal Infirmary, Department of Cytology, Barrack Road, Dundee

**Professor D. B. Fournier**
> Aerztlicher Direkton, ABT 8.1.4., Gun-Geburtsh Radiologie, Universitaets Frauenklinik, Vobstrasse 9, D-6900, Heidelberg, Germany

**Professor R. Goebel**
> Chefarzt der Frauenklinik, Evangelis ches Krankenhaus, Virchowstrasse 20, D-2400, Oberhsausen, Germany

**Professor A. Gorins**
> 20 Rue Clement Marot, 75008 Paris, France

**Mr C. P. Hinton FRCS**
Surgical Research Registrar, City Hospital, Hucknall Road, Nottingham,
NG5 1PD

**Dr H. Junkermann**
Universitaets Frauenklinik, Vobstrasse 9, D-6900, Heidelberg, Germany

**Mr M. Kissin FRCS**
Research Fellow, Chester Beatty Institute of Cancer Research, Fulham
Road, London

**Professor G. Leyendecker**
Universitaets-Frauenklinik, Benusberg, D-5300 Bonn, Germany

**Mr R. Mansel FRCS**

Department of Medicine, Division of Oncology, University of Texas,
Health Science Center at San Antonio, 7703 Floyd Curl Drive, San
Antonio, Texas

**Dr G. Potts**
Sterling Winthrop Research Institute, Columbia Turnpike, Rensselaer NY
12144

**Mr D. Preece FRCS**
Department of Surgery, Ninewalls Hospital, Dundee, Scotland DD1 9SY

**Dr G. Rannevik**
Fertility Research Institute, Limhammnsvagen, 42 217 74, Malmo,
Sweden

**Dr Th Rasmussen**
Rontgen afd, Hjorring Hospital 9800, Hjorring, Denmark

**Professor N. B. Shaikh**
Consultant Surgeon, University Coll Hospital, Surgical Unit, Gower
Street, London WC1E 6AU

**Dr T. Tobiassen**
Gyn afd, Hjorring Hospital, 9800 Hjorring, Denmark

**Mr P. Walsh FRCS**
University Department of Surgery, Royal Liverpool Hospital, PO Box
147, Liverpool L69 3BX

*PARTICIPANTS*
**Mr E. A. Benson FRCS**
Leeds General Infirmary, Great George Street, Leeds 1, West Yorkshire

**Dr Eggert-Kruse**
University Gynaecology Clinic, Heidelberg, W. Germany

**Mr D. F. Fossard FRCS**
Royal Infirmary, Leicester

**Professor W. D. George**
Western Infirmary, Glasgow G11 6NT

**Mr J. R. W. Gumpert FRCS**
> *Department of Surgery, Royal Sussex County Hospital, Brighton, Sussex*

**Dr U. Hermann**
> *Berne, Switzerland*

**Mr S. Kumar FRCS**
> *University Hospital of Wales, Cardiff, Wales*

**Mr E. C. G. Lee FRCS**
> *John Radcliffe Hospital, Oxford*

**Mr S. J. Leinster FRCS**
> *University Department of Surgery, PO Box 147, Liverpool*

**Mr K. Lloyd-Williams FRCS**
> *Department of Surgery, Royal United Hospital, Combe Park, Bath, Avon*

**Mr J. M. Morrison FRCS**
> *Selly Oak Hospital, Birmingham 29 6JD*

**Professor N. O'Higgins**
> *St Vincent's Hospital, Elm Park, Dublin 4, Ireland*

**Mr S. P. Parbhoo FRCS**
> *Academic Department of Surgery, Royal Free Hospital, Pond Street, London NW3*

**Mr M. Perry FRCS**
> *Queen Alexandra Hospital, Portsmouth, Hants PO6 3LY*

**Mr S. J. A. Powis FRCS**
> *Northampton General Hospital, Northampton*

**Mr P. H. Powley FRCS**
> *Princess Margaret Hospital, Okus Road, Swindon*

**Mr J. Rickett FRCS**
> *Torbay Hospital, Torquay, Devon*

**Mr G. T. Watts FRCS**
> *General Hospital, Birmingham*

# Contents

# Session 1:
# National differences in nomenclature and approach to benign breast disease

## CHAIRMAN'S INTRODUCTION

**L. E. HUGHES**

*University Department of Surgery,*
*Welsh National School of Medicine,*
*Cardiff, Wales*

The first session of this symposium deals with nomenclature and approach—a subject well chosen because benign breast disease is an area of great confusion. Although confusion is not unusual in surgery, it is certainly more common with BBD (as it is known in Cardiff) than in many other surgical fields. Why has this come about? I think to some extent because we have been frustrated by the limited number and scope of the tools available to us to study the disease, at least until recent years.

A number of great names stand out in the field of benign breast disease surgery— Schimmelbusch in Germany, Geshichter in America, Semb in Norway, Hedley Atkins in Britain and one perhaps not so often recognized, the late Sir Alan Parkes, who did very important work in breast disease before turning his interests elsewhere. Each of these people tended to start off from scratch; they did their own work and presented it and then sooner or later someone else would take it up. Each time there was a tendency for different nomenclature to be used, and although each worker added to our knowledge they also added to our confusion by producing yet another nomenclature.

I have never before thought of these confusing differences in nomenclature in national terms, and I find this a very interesting concept. In this first session we have four contributors talking about nomenclature and approach to the disease from a national as well as from an overall viewpoint.

*Benign Breast Disease, Edited by M. Baum, W. D. George, and L. E. Hughes, 1985: Royal Society of Medicine International Congress and Symposia series No. 76, published by The Royal Society of Medicine.*

# Nomenclature of benign breast disease, with particular reference to national differences in approach

**P. E. PREECE**

*Ninewells Hospital and Medical School,
University of Dundee, Scotland, UK*

Benign breast disease, more than any other area of clinical practice in medicine, would appear to have been bedevilled by confusing terminology. When a variety of treatments is used for a single condition, this usually means that the optimal therapy is unknown. By the same token, when there is a multiplicity of names for a single condition, it can be inferred that the best name is not available because the pathogenesis is unknown or in dispute.

Apart from the different terms used in the different countries where these conditions are observed, the most important reason for the confusing terminology for benign breast diseases which exists today is ignorance of their aetiology. Another contributory factor has been uncritical adoption of terms across specialty boundaries, with no great regard for their precise original meeting. One example is the use of the word 'dysplasia' (a morphological term for well-accepted cellular changes which are usually irreversible) applied to certain radiological appearances of the breast which are of uncertain significance and which, if biopsied, rarely show dysplasia as defined histopathologically.

One aspect of benign breast disease about which there is little argument is that this term embraces a wide range of clinical, radiological and pathological entities. It seems to me that a prerequisite to a discussion on nomenclature is a working classification. Ideally any such classification should be useful to all the parties with an interest in the condition. I suggest there are at least six of these: the patient, the general practitioner, the surgeon, the physician, the pathologist and the radiologist. For benign breast disease of females, it is possible to construct a clinical classification which embraces the normal life-span. This provides an easy *aide-memoire* which, with a few additions, is fairly comprehensive. What this scheme, shown in Table 1, lacks in chronological accuracy it makes up for in memorability for it can be thought of as the 'Seven Benign Ages of Woman'.

The 'neonatal developmental conditions' are the subareolar lumps palpated at birth due to stimulation from maternal sex hormones (misnamed mastitis neonátorum) and neonatal breast abscess.

'Peripubertal developmental conditions' include the solitary lump which often

*Benign Breast Disease, Edited by M. Baum, W. D. George, and L. E. Hughes, 1985: Royal Society of Medicine International Congress and Symposia series No. 76, published by The Royal Society of Medicine.*

*Table 1*
*Clinical classification*

| | |
|---|---|
| Neonatal ⎫ Peripubertal ⎬ | Developmental conditions |
| Youth | Benign tumours |
| Young adulthood | Benign painful lumpiness |
| Reproductive phase | Disorders of lactation |
| Late premenopausal | Cystic disease |
| Perimenopausal | Duct ectasia/periductal mastitis |

appears deep to the areola just before any other signs of puberty are seen, and congenital absence or retraction of nipple and polymasia. In 'youth', that is the first few years after the breasts have developed, fibroadenoma is common. For completeness, intraduct papilloma can be considered here, there being little disagreement that this lesion is benign.

In 'young adulthood' benign, painful lumpiness, perhaps currently known in the UK as mastopathy, is the benign breast disease about which there is the greatest divergence of opinion in both nomenclature and approach. It must be conceded that it is not confined to young adulthood, but it will not be contested that it is only seen during reproductive life, that is, in premenopausal women. In the context of this symposium, it is this condition, whatever we choose to call it, to which we shall be directing much of our attention. Its catalogue of synonyms, with their 'pros' and 'cons' are best considered later.

The 'reproductive phase' of female life is, of course, in practice, highly variable for different individuals in terms of actual age. By this, I mean time spent pregnant and lactating. During this phase, we see fissure of the nipple, milk fever, puerperal breast abscess and galactocele. 'Late premenopausal' is the last 10 years or so before menstruation ceases, normally the years between the ages of 40 and 50. These are, for the most part, the years when cysts occur.

The least satisfactory component of this Shakespearean parody is my last one, the seventh age, which I have called 'perimenopausal', and to which I have allocated the duct ectasia/periductal mastitis spectrum of disorders. These conditions, also known in English-speaking countries as comedo-mastitis and plasma-cell mastitis may, in my experience, manifest at any time in adult life, even well after the menopause. They can give rise, as probably will be shown later in this symposium, to any and all of the local breast symptoms which occur, namely, lump, nipple retraction, nipple discharge, eczema and pain.

The first term to discuss, if only to deprecate and dismiss, is the root 'cyst' which has so frequently figured inappropriately in the nomenclature of benign breast disease, both in the clinic and in the laboratory. Common examples are 'cystic mastitis' and 'fibrocystic disease'. In the scheme suggested as a catalogue for benign breast disease it was noted that cysts occur almost exclusively in the last 10 years of reproductive life, certainly as far as their clinical manifestations are concerned. Since cysts are so easily diagnosed, any breast disease which these accompany can simply be annotated 'with cysts' and all the cyst-bearing adjectives can be withdrawn from circulation, so giving a simpler currency for negotiating the problems of aetiology.

To return now to the entity I have, for simplicity, called 'benign painful lumpiness': this is a complaint which often occurs in young adulthood, but, as already mentioned, it is not strictly confined to that phase of life. The patients with this condition describe two symptoms: pain and lumpiness. Characteristically it is often worse in the days before a period, often cyclical, with the onset of the period sometimes relieving the symptoms. Both breasts are frequently affected (in a series from Cardiff 50 per cent of patients were simultaneously affected in both breasts) and the parts of the breast most frequently involved are the upper and outer quadrants.

One of the earliest used terms for this is to be found in the French literature. It is '*induration en masse*', a term used in the first half of the last century (Velpeau 1856), and one which would seem more appropriate and greatly superior to a number of words which were used later. Velpeau specified the age-incidence of '*induration en masse*' as 25–40 years. An 1856 English translation of his description is interesting:

'Clinically, there is induration of a part or the whole of the gland. Usually this is only fully appreciated by comparison of the affected part of the breast with the opposite. It is occasionally accompanied by lancinating, deep-seated and dull pain. The gland appears lumpy without manifest increase in size, and there is no indication of its being the seat of the least engorgement or inflammation. It is a difficult condition to differentiate from breast cancer. The importance of distinguishing it from this is self-evident.'

About the same time, and perhaps inspired by this same source, a Jacksonian prize winner at the Royal College of Surgeons of England (Birkett 1850) described a painful state of the breast as 'mazodynia', and distinguished two classes, *with* and *without* 'induration'. Rather along the same lines, considering pain as the dominant symptom, Theodor Billroth in Germany defined three categories of 'neuralgia of the breast glands' (Billroth 1879). They were: those with discrete tumours, granular breast and those with no palpable abnormality. The term 'mastitis' came into vogue towards the end of the 19th century, to describe painful, lumpy breasts. Even then, a voice was raised questioning this usage, in a paper published in the *Boston Medical and Surgical Journal* of 1900 (Cabot 1900). The author was the first of several clinicians to advocate more precise terminology. At that time in continental Europe, the problem was partly resolved by the use of eponyms. Thus in France, '*maladie de Reclus*' was used (devised, I believe, from the name of a surgeon Paul Reclus, rather than the word '*reclus*' meaning recluse, with its implications of nulliparity and spinsterhood). In 1931 the American pathologist Max Cutler described the use of the term 'mastitis' for painful lumpy breasts as 'obviously erroneous' (Cutler 1931). Twenty years later, no less an authority on the breast disease than the late Mr David Patey, referring to the benign breast disease called 'chronic mastitis', in a lecture to medical students said:

'By almost universal consent, chronic organismal inflammation and the aseptic inflammatory conditions referred to as "periductal" or "plasma-cell mastitis" are excluded.'

He went on to show that cystic disease of the breast is not mastitis and concluded:

'The term chronic mastitis is the expression of an attempt to define in terms of organic disease a *symptom*—pain in the breast. Analysis shows this attempt to be unsatisfactory.'

If the nomenclature which was derived by clinicians is 'questionable', 'unsatisfactory', even 'obviously erroneous', have the pathologists done any better? In 1928, Carl Semb specified a subgroup of benign breast diseases which included localized foci of painful lumpiness as 'fibroadenomatosis simplex'. The rather similar term 'adenofibrosis' was applied to the same morphology, namely proliferation of the connective tissue of the breast, which appeared to have compressed and scattered the small ducts and acini which had also, frequently, undergone proliferation themselves. The word 'adenosis' derived from Scotland, where it was introduced into the literature by Mrs E. K. Dawson of Edinburgh, who used it for epithelial proliferation within the secretory part of the mammary gland and so evolved the word 'fibroadenosis' (Dawson 1933). It has been used in both clinical and pathological contexts, frequently as a clinical term when no biopsy has been required, and as a pathological term when no proliferation of acinar epithelium is in fact present. One other term which was suggested for the same entity was 'mazoplasia'. Coined in America (Cheatle and Cutler 1931) this term has not been widely used in Britain and rarely figures in English language literature from other countries. It means literally 'much growth' referring to hyperplasia of both connective tissue and acini.

Currently, both the majority of clinicians and the majority of pathologists who deal with benign breast disease are realizing that there is no rigid correlation between the clinical presentation and the microscopic appearances of these conditions. Most recognize also that much still requires to be known and understood about their aetiology, evolution and natural history. As a first step towards discovering these things a simplified nomenclature which was internationally acceptable, yet flexible, would be a useful contribution. The basic requirement for such a nomenclature would be that it respected the precise original meaning of the root words coined, and that these root words implied no more about aetiology than could be reasonably supported by the evidence available at any given time.

# References

Billroth, T. (1879). In *Handbook of women's disease*, Vol. 2, p. 35. F. Enke, Stuttgart.
Birkett, J. (1850). In *The diseases of the breast and their treatment*, p. 164. Longman, Brown, Green & Longman, London.
Cabot, R. C. (1900). *Boston Med. Surg. J.*, **143**, 555.
Cheatle, G. L. and Cutler, M. (1931). In *Tumours of the breast*, p. 77. Edward Arnold, London.
Cutler, M. (1931). *J. Amer. Med. Assoc.*, **96**, 1201.
Dawson, E. K. (1933). *Edinb. Med. J.*, **40**, 57.

# A useful clinical classification of benign breast disease

**H. JUNKERMANN, W. EGGERT-KRUSE, J. TEUBNER, F. KUBLI AND D. V. FOURNIER**

*University Gynaecology Clinic and German Cancer Research Centre, Heidelberg, West Germany*

We use the term 'mastopathy' for a clinical syndrome of benign breast lesions, which is characterized by increased nodularity, pain and, eventually, pathological secretion. This syndrome is usually found in women between the ages of 30 and 50 years; after the menopause the complaints usually subside. Clinically we found the syndrome of mastopathy in 21 per cent of 6000 unselected patients who consulted us for reasons other than breast complaints. Histologically, mastopathy was found in 53 per cent of unselected women in post mortem studies by Frantz *et al.* (1951).

Imbalance of oestrogens and gestagens with an oestrogen dominance seems to be the cause of mastopathy, but the exact nature of this imbalance is still controversial. Although latent hyperprolactinaemia has been found in women with benign breast diseases, the causal relationship of the disease remains unclear. Mild thyroid dysfunction of the same type as that found in endemic goitre has recently been found in a high percentage of cases by Peters *et al.* (1981). Other hormones, such as corticoids, growth hormone, insulin and androgens, also have an influence on breast tissue, but nothing is known about their significance in the development of mastopathy.

The rather poorly defined clinical syndrome of mastopathy is to be contrasted with a clear histological definition, which should also be used clinically as far as possible. Bässler (1978) defines three forms of mastopathy: mastopathy cystica fibrosa, fibrosis mammae, and mastodynia/mazoplasia. The most important form quantitively is mastopathy cystica fibrosa.

Histologically, we find in mastopathy a combination of abnormalities which are either of a progressive or a regressive nature. Progressive changes, perhaps currently described as mastopathy in the UK, are adenosis, papillomatosis or cystadenosis, while regressive changes are cystic involution or fibroadenomatosis.

In the case of gross cystic disease shown in Fig. 1, opacities with a clearly defined margin can be seen. Radiologically, we are not able to distinguish between cystic or

**Figures in this paper are to be found in the colour section at the end of the symposia.**

*Benign Breast Disease, Edited by M. Baum, W. D. George, and L. E. Hughes, 1985: Royal Society of Medicine International Congress and Symposia series No. 76, published by The Royal Society of Medicine.*

solid lesions. Ultrasonographically, multiple large cysts with a diameter of several centimetres can be demonstrated in both breasts (Fig. 2).

In another patient (Fig. 3) several rounded structures can be seen in the left breast but it is not possible to tell whether these are cysts or solid tumours. Sonographically, a cyst can be demonstrated at (1), however with no echoes from within it (Fig. 4). Reflex enhancement behind the cyst can be seen with lateral attenuation. In contrast, at (2) a tumour was found with homogenous reflexes which corresponds to a fibroadenoma.

In mastopathy, the mammogram is often so dense that its assessment becomes unreliable. In the case shown in Fig. 5, a radiological and clinical diagnosis of benign mastopathy was made, but sonography (Fig. 6) disclosed a 1 cm carcinoma.

An important controversial question is the risk of development of cancer in women with benign breast disease. According to Bässler (1978) the important question is whether intraductal epithelial proliferations exist and whether these proliferations contain atypical cells. He describes three groups: mastopathia cystica fibrosa without intraductal epithelial proliferation, mastopathia cystica fibrosa with epithelial proliferation but without atypical cells, and mastopathia cystica fibrosa with epithelial proliferation with atypical cells. In group I, with no epithelial proliferation (about 70 per cent of biopsy specimens), no increased risk of cancer is apparent. In group II (21 per cent of biopsy specimens), there is a slight increase in cancer risk. A variety of different benign breast disorders exists which are often found as part of mastopathia cystica fibrosa. Each of these disorders may also exist as a disease on its own.

Sclerosing adenosis is defined as a proliferation of myoepithelial cells. It is often found in fibrocystic mastopathy. Radiologically, it can be defined by its characteristic calcification pattern. Sclerosing adenosis does not carry a cancer risk.

Fibroadenoma develops from the hormonally responsive mantle tissue and is usually found in younger women. Radiologically, fibroadenoma cannot be differentiated from cysts. No cancer risk exists.

Papillary adenomata are usually detected by serous or bloody discharge from the nipple. They are mostly found in older, often postmenopausal, women. Singular papillomas do not carry an increased cancer risk, though diffuse papillomatosis is considered a risk factor for mammary carcinoma. Duct ectasia, caused by retention of secretory debris in the duct system, is also found in older women. This lesión also carries no cancer risk.

The heterogeneous response of the breast to hormonal stimulation, and the range of reactions produced in different parts of the same breast, may give rise to considerable error even in the histological classification of benign breast diseases. Furthermore, in cases of subcutaneous mastectomy, with different methods of specimen preparation, different numbers of premalignant and malignant changes can be found.

The lack of agreement on classification of different forms of mastopathy, whether clinical, paraclinical or histological methods are used, together with the problem of differentiating mastopathy from the range of normal breast conditions, has led us to propose our own simple classification based on clinical and paraclinical criteria.

We have defined as mild mastopathy, slight radiological dysplasia with no evidence of proliferative changes, and clinically only slight induration or nodularity, but with pronounced premenstrual engorgement. Thermography is only abnormal premenstrually and the leading complaint of the patient is premenstrual mastodynia, which can be considered as one symptom of the premenstrual syndrome. In mild mastopathy no diagnositic difficulties exist.

We classify as severe mastopathy, pronounced radiological dysplasia with evidence of proliferation, and, particularly, microcalcifications, clinically pronounced induration or nodularity which impairs clinical assessment. Thermography is also postmenstrually abnormal. Mastodynia may exist throughout the cycle, though it is usually premenstrually pronounced. Mastodynia does not exist in all cases. The leading complaint of the patient is either the mastodynia or the increased nodularity which causes diagnostic uncertainty.

## References

Bässler, R. (1978). In *Spezielle pathologische Anatomie* (eds Doerr, Seifer and Uehlinger), Vol. 11. Springer, Berlin.
Frantz, V. K., *et al.* (1951). *Cancer*, **4**, 762–83.
Peters, F., *et al.* (1981). *Wochenschr.*, **59**, 403–7.

# Benign mastopathy: classification and epidemiology. A practical approach to benign breast disease in France

## S. LARUE-CHARLUS AND A. JM. AUDEBERT

*Institut Aquitain de Recherche et d'Etude en Reproduction Humaine,
40 Cour de Verdun, Bordeaux, France*

Cases of benign breast disease are extremely common and require an accurate diagnosis to be made, not least to relieve the patient of her anxieties.

Because of the underlying fear of malignancy, the task of the specialist breast centre involves the detection, recognition and investigation of the two types of benign breast disease—pre-neoplastic lesions, which warrant radical treatment, and proliferative lesions which require preventive treatment.

Benign breast diseases are divided into two large categories, depending on the starting point of the histological anomaly—the milk duct or the lobule (de Brux 1982):

(a) *Milk duct*  Tissue proliferations at the level of the interlobular milk duct represent the classical dendritic adenoma. Two types of lesion are recognized—isolated intragalactophoric papilloma and the rarer multiple papillomatosis, usually multifocal with lesions frequently at the boundary of malignancy.

(b) *Lobule*  Proliferations of the lobular endings are much more common and varied; they may be 'pure' or 'mixed'. In the case of pure proliferations, distinction is made between hyperplasia of the diffuse lobules (adenosis) and the well-limited tumour (adenoma or adenofibroma, its developed form). Proliferations may be mixed either with hyperplasia of the myoepithelial cells (sclerosising adenosis, invasive adenosclerosis), or with hyperplasia of the connective tissue (fibroadenoma, phyllode tumour).

To these can be added, on the one hand, a complex of these different forms and, on the other, physiological degeneration of the mammary gland, more a fibrosclerosis than a lipomatosis, causing classical sclerocystic disease of the breast.

Within the framework of this histological classification a section should be reserved for the evolutive or intermediate forms. These are cases of benign mastopathy with atypical hyperplasia, the cellular type being located either at the milk duct or the lobule. These lesions are promoted by hyperoestrogenism, that is, an oestro-

*Benign Breast Disease, Edited by M. Baum, W. D. George, and L. E. Hughes, 1985: Royal Society of Medicine International Congress and Symposia series No. 76, published by The Royal Society of Medicine.*

progestational imbalance. Atypical papillary hyperplasia may be involved, filling one milk duct, with all the intermediate forms, depending on the cellular atypia, leading to malignant hyperplasias. Atypical lobular hyperplasias (Haagensen 1971) fill the lobule–milk duct junction. They display the same intermediate forms but are likely to be multifocal.

Whatever the case, these hyperplasias are not accompanied by palpable tumour and it is important to remember that they may coexist with invasive cancer.

The evolutive aspects of mastopathy are very important but the chapter has scarcely been opened; many studies, notably multicentric work, are still in progress.

Several publications note the presence of benign breast lesions in 35–40 per cent of sections removed at mastectomy because of cancer (Contesso et al. 1975). These figures, however, are very close to the percentage of breast lesions discovered on systematic examination of autopsy sections of the breasts of women who had not died from breast disease. However, various studies have shown that the risk of cancer is increased twofold in cases of cystic disease, sixfold in cases of atypical hyperplasia (Page et al. 1978) and 14-fold if an hereditary factor is additionally present (Haagensen 1971). In these retrospective studies the lesion removed cannot have degenerated and so the problem is one of relationships or coexistence and thus of the surrounding environment with promoting factors.

Assay of the biochemical cellular components which give information on the hormone receptors and enzymatic activity will, in the near future, enable recognition of the degree of cellular differentiation, the rate of cellular growth and the metastatic potential, in other words, the exact profile of the development of the lesion (Martin 1982; Pichon et al. 1982).

## Epidemiology—incidence in the population

The results of even the most important studies on the incidence of benign breast disease are invalidated when they are concerned only with patients who had undergone surgery (Cole et al. 1978). In the United States, benign breast disease was found in 1·3 per thousand of which fibrocystic disease accounts for 0·9 per thousand and adenofibroma for 0·33 per thousand. Other studies which included patients consulting because of benign breast disease (not just those who had undergone surgery or biopsy) give an incidence some 20 per cent higher (Brinton et al. 1981).

The incidence curves differ greatly between the two histological types; for adenofibroma, the maximum incidence is at 30 years, whilst for fibrocystic disease the maximum is at age 45 (Bremond 1982). The incidence curve for breast cancer is also different, growing progressively higher from 30 to 70 years, with a slight plateau at 55.

## Risk factors

The epidemiology of benign breast disease is a very recent concept, especially in France. Marital status, parity, age at first pregnancy and lactation have no effect either on the risk or on the incidence of benign breast disease (Bremond 1982). Precocious puberty has no effect but late menopause increases the incidence of fibrocystic disease.

Socio-economic levels do not affect the risk, but it should be noted that the use of medical resources is not the same at all socio-economic levels. A family history of cancer does not increase the risk of the benign mastopathies.

Although food and stress affect the incidence, obesity would appear to protect against benign breast disease (Brinton et al. 1981).

Finally, hormonal factors, as in the case of neoplastic lesions, play a very important role. There is no increase in circulating oestrogens in cases of benign mastopathy, but very often a luteal insufficiency is present (Sitruk-Ware *et al.* 1979) and prolactin levels may vary greatly. Corrective measures should be taken.

## Iatrogenic factors

Iatrogenic factors relate essentially to hormone replacement therapy and the use of oral contraceptive agents.

In effect, retrospective studies of oestroprogestogens are invalid when they involve benign breast disease patients who have been subjected to surgery. These eliminate cases of functional symptomatology without aetiological proof and take into account neither possible improvements brought about by oestroprogestogens nor deteriorations which may have caused treatment to be stopped. Neither do these studies take into account case histories which constitute a contraindication to treatment. It must also be noted that most of the studies—certainly those that began 10 or more years ago—involved products given in higher hormone dosage than is now the case. However, it is clear that oestroprogestogen oral contraceptives reduce the incidence of benign breast disease, by about 20 per cent if all authors are considered, the protection effect either ceasing when treatment is stopped (Vessey *et al.* 1972) or continuing for several years (Ory *et al.* 1976).

Almost the same criticism can be made about studies of oestrogen alone. There are no trials comparing different oestrogens or different dosages in relation to age and route of administration; the starting point of the studies has always been surgery and a history of benign breast disease has been a contraindication to treatment. However, the risk certainly does exist: the incidence of mastopathy increases if the user of oestrogens exceeds four years (Nomura and Comstock 1976). The risk also increases with age (perimenopause), past history of benign breast disease and where there has been a previous hormone imbalance.

## Risk of cancer and benign breast disease

The relationship between mastopathies and cancer is weak but real. Eight per cent of women undergoing surgery for benign breast disease will suffer from cancer (Ernster 1981). However, the incidence varies as a function of the histological type. Although the incidence of cancer does not increase in those women suffering from adenofibroma, it does in those with epithelial hyperplasia and still more in cases of cellular atypia.

After five years of oral contraceptive use, a past history of benign breast disease multiplies the risk of cancer by a factor of eight (Fasal and Paffen Barger 1975) and, although a past history of benign mastopathy alone multiplies the risk by only two, if oestrogen therapy is added the risk factor is increased to seven (Hoover *et al.* 1976).

## Detection

The detection of mastopathies consists essentially of recognizing the intermediate forms which lead towards breast cancer. It is based on: (*a*) research into risk factors; (*b*) determination of criteria of evolution (clinical, radiological and ultrasound); (*c*) reliable and repeated cytology; (*d*) assays of hormone receptors and cellular enzymatic activity. Thus it becomes possible to distinguish between the mastopathies which are likely to lead to cancer and those which represent a 'signal-symptom' of hormonal imbalance—itself a carcinogenetic risk factor.

In France, the diagnosis and treatment of benign breast diseases take place at three different levels: first, at the few specialized centres which have now been opened, and at the anti-cancer out-patient departments and the obstetric and gynaecology departments which have a special section for breast disease; second, by the gynaecologist and general practitioner during consultation, notably for contraception advice (and this emphasizes the need for specialized postgraduate training). Third is the detection of the condition by the patient through self-examination, a technique which is still in an early educational phase.

Detection, based mainly on this classical 'cyto-radio-clinico' tripod, incurs an error of below 0·25 per cent when all results converge.

In summary, then, epidemiology of the benign breast diseases constitutes part of the epidemiology of breast cancer. That alone justifies its study and no longer can mastodynia and other manifestations of benign breast disease be considered inconsequential conditions connected with the patient's female status.

## References

Bremond, A. (1982). In *Mastopathies benignes*. Masson, Paris.
Brinton, L. A., *et al.* (1981). *Amer. J. Epidemiol.,* **113**, 203.
de Brux, J. (1982). In *Mastopathies benignes*. Masson, Paris.
Cole, P., *et al.* (1978). *Amer. J. Epidemiol.,* **108**, 112.
Contesso, G., *et al.* (1975). *J. Gynaec. Obstet. Biol. Reprod.,* **4**, 5–20.
Ernster, V. L. (1981). *Epidemiol. Rev.,* **2**, 194–202.
Fasal, E., and Paffen Barger, P. S. (1975). *J. Natl Cancer Inst.,* **55**, 767.
Haagensen, C. D. (1971). In *Diseases of the breast*. W. B. Saunders, Philadelphia.
Hoover, R., *et al.* (1976). *New Engl. J. Med.,* **295**, 401.
Martin, P. M. (1982). In *Mastopathies bénignes*. Masson, Paris.
Nomura, A., and Comstock. G. W. (1976). *Amer. J. Epidemiol.,* **103**, 439.
Ory, H., *et al.* (1976). *New Engl. J. Med.,* **294**, 419.
Page, D., *et al.* (1978). *J. Natl Cancer Inst.* **61**, 1055–63.
Pichon, M. F., *et al.* (1982). In *Mastopathies bénignes*. Masson, Paris.
Sitruk-Ware, R., *et al.* (1979). *Obstet. Gynecol.* **53**, 457–60.
Vessey, M. P., *et al.* (1972). *Brit. Med. J.* **3**, 719.

# The terminology of benign breast disease in Scandinavia

## TH. RASMUSSEN

*Department of Radiodiagnostics,*
*Hjørring County Hospital, Hjørring, Denmark*

For clinical rather than research purposes, the nomenclature of benign breast diseases is very much simplified in Scandinavia (Table 1) and yet it is easy to incorporate the mammographic findings into the clinical terminology.

*Table 1*
*Benign breast disease nomenclature in Scandinavia*

| | |
|---|---|
| Traumatic | Fat necrosis |
| Infectious | Acute mastitis (puerperal and non-puerperal); abscess |
| Tumours | Intraductal papilloma; fibroadenoma |
| Fibrocystic disease | Fibroadenosis, with or without cysts |

It will be seen from Table 1 that intraductal papilloma is considered to be a benign condition for which surgery is certainly not always indicated. Galactographic and mammographic control of the growth is, however, necessary. The benign nature of fibroadenomata is always confirmed by adenography and mammography as well as by thin-needle aspiration. The indications for surgery differ according to the site, the rate of growth and the primary size.

What in the UK is known as fibrocystic disease, in Scandinavia is called fibroadenosis, with or without cysts (Table 2). We consider this disease to be a progressive benign process, starting at age 20–30 years, with lobular localized or diffuse adenosis, our name for glandular hyperplasia. Fibrosis develops later. In severe cases, it may manifest itself as sclerosing adenosis.

In some patients duct ectasia develops. This may become severe, with diffuse spread and almost invariably associated with the development of cysts. For mammographic purposes, cysts of less than 1 cm in size are known as microcysts; larger cysts (1 cm or more) are called macrocysts. Duct ectasia with cysts is nearly always followed by

*Benign Breast Disease, Edited by M. Baum, W. D. George, and L. E. Hughes, 1985: Royal Society of Medicine International Congress and Symposia series No. 76, published by The Royal Society of Medicine.*

Table 2

Fibrocystic disease: Scandinavian terminology

| Adenosis + ↓ | Fibrosis (sclerosing adenosis) |
| | Duct ectasia (and secretory disease) |
| | Small cysts |
| | Few localized |
| | Massive diffuse spread |
| | large cysts (≥ 1 cm)—palpable as tumours |

secretory disease. Spontaneous secretion is rare, but slight pressure on the ampulla usually produces secretion. We have found that the colour of the secretion depends upon the duration of the disease and upon the number and size of the cysts. It may thus vary from light-milky to blue-black or green in the most severe cases.

Macrocysts may develop at all stages of fibrocystic disease. Their development appears to depend rather more upon the presence of heavy glandular structure than upon the number and spread of microcysts.

Finally, we are fully aware that the term 'fibrocystic breast disease' is so widely accepted that any attempt to replace it may be futile. However, we think it unfortunate that the term in no way indicates the adenoid tissue which, after all, is the prime target for hormonal stimulation. In Scandinavia, therefore, we shall probably continue to speak of 'fibroadenosis, with or without cysts'.

# Session 1:

## CHAIRMAN'S SUMMARY

### L. E. HUGHES

*University Department of Surgery,*
*Welsh National School of Medicine,*
*Cardiff, Wales*

We've seen from these four presentations, from four different countries, that there are many similarities in approach but also refreshing differences in emphasis. The papers were certainly complementary to each other in a somewhat surprising way.

Paul Preece stressed the clinical details of painful lumpiness as part of a process which can be classified on an age basis, and I think that is a very interesting concept.

Dr Junkermann stressed the relationship to normality—21 per cent of patients from a normal population have clinical abnormality, and 50 per cent of 'normal' patients have histological changes. He laid particular emphasis on the German view of the histology and pathogenesis, and stressed also that element of benign breast disease which may be on the pathway towards cancer. He classified benign breast disease as slight (which I think we would find easier to follow than 'light') and severe.

Dr Larue-Charlus brought in the importance of both epithelium and stroma—so often we forget the importance of stroma, but it is just as much under hormonal influence as the epithelium and perhaps we get into trouble as often as we do because we don't take the stroma into account. And then he raised particularly the spectre of cancer which hangs over every patient with benign breast disease and the very important concept of additive risk factors in patients who may develop cancer. He went on to stress the fallacies which arise from the limitations of our investigations and why we have so many different 'answers' to some of the problems.

Finally, Dr Rasmussen stressed the importance of a simple approach, and that was a very refreshing way to end up. He also brought to our attention the importance of radiology, not only in diagnosis and treatment but also to our understanding of benign breast disease, where it has made an enormous contribution; we would do well to remember that. The other point that came out of the work in Denmark was that this is an evolving process; it is continuous throughout the patient's reproductive life and many of the conditions evolve one from another.

Perhaps we can leave it with a suggestion that there are three processes: first, the disorders of the normal physiological processes of the breast, that's development in the first 10–15 years of the reproductive life and involution in the last 10–15 years; the second group consists of those with duct ectasia and periductal mastitis which certainly have a specific histology, which suggests some primary immune attack on

*Benign Breast Disease, Edited by M. Baum, W. D. George, and L. E. Hughes, 1985: Royal Society of Medicine International Congress and Symposia series No. 76, published by The Royal Society of Medicine.*

the ducts; and then the third group is the cancer-related conditions, the processes that are premalignant. I wonder whether we can put any of those together, except that they are often coincidental?

If we look at the disorders of development and involution, in the first 15 years we have the fibroadenoma when both epithelium and stroma are involved; we have the duct papilloma when epithelium alone is involved; and perhaps they can be regarded as developmental disorders and not neoplastic.

When we come to the middle-aged group, we have this diffuse area of (I hardly know what to call it after the four papers) hormonal mastopathy—a terrible term—with or without cysts, or perhaps fibroadenosis, because that certainly, with or without cysts, is a very good term. I think we would do well to get a uniform term for that group—the biggest group—indicating with or without cysts, with or without pain. Perhaps we will get somewhere with it.

And then the involutional phase: the lobules are regressing, the epithelium is regressing, that very specialized hormonal-sensitive connective tissue of the lobule is replaced by fibrous tissue; things get out of relationship, and the cysts form. There is cystic degeneration rather than the normal lobular involution and if there is too much fibrosis you get sclerosing adenosis. Then one needs a second group which will cover duct ectasia and periductal mastitis, whether it is a result of obstruction; or of progestogen causing relaxation of ducts; or of an immune attack on the ducts which then destroys the muscle; who knows? But we have to cover also the cases of periductal mastitis which occur in the first 10 years of reproductive life, because recurrent subareolar abscess can be seen in single girls of 15 or 16 as well as in the larger group in the perimenopausal age group.

And then, the third group, the cancer group: I think the message is that these cases are different. The cancer risks may be coincidental with the other aspects of benign mastopathy. Probably the two do go hand in hand to some extent, but we must define specific cancer risk factors rather than talk about the cancer risks of hormonal mastopathy.

Now I would like to throw the session open for discussion.

# Discussion: Session 1

**Hughes**

I would like to put a question to Dr Rasmussen. I was interested to see that you put duct ectasia and periductal mastitis in the overall group of fibrocystic disease. Do you feel strongly about this?

**Rasmussen**

Yes, I do. We have seen duct ectasia, not in the premenopausal woman, but very early in the 30s, and we find some connection with the number of breast feedings and the abrupt cessation of breast feeding. This results in duct ectasia which later on becomes more pronounced and leads to small cysts. It's progressive. But you have to look for the secretion with light pressure—there's no spontaneous secretion.

**Junkermann**

This seems to me to be a very interesting concept. I understand what you say about abrupt cessation of breast feeding possibly causing duct ectasia, but the concept that the duct ectasia persists for a long period of time is quite contrary to what is thought in Germany; I would have thought that with monthly breast changes this duct ectasia would resolve after a short time—just as galactarrhoea often resolves spontaneously.

**Lee**

I'd like to make a number of points. First, from the papers, it didn't seem to be clear that most of the points are still controversial, and this, I feel, is a matter of importance. For instance, we have just heard a discussion about duct ectasia and the same could be said for a number of different instances where evidence was presented without giving the full range from both sides. I'd like to stress the point that in benign breast disease the epidemological studies are very deficient at the moment and we certainly don't have all the data. These are studies we should all be doing if we can.

My second point is that I was particularly interested in the idea of a symposium on nomenclature, because that seems to be the most crucial thing for all of us at the moment; we are all speaking a different language and a different science. However, I don't think the speakers covered this problem adequately.

*Benign Breast Disease*, Edited by *M. Baum, W. D. George, and L. E. Hughes, 1985: Royal Society of Medicine International Congress and Symposia series No. 76, published by The Royal Society of Medicine.*

I was particularly interested in Mr Preece's paper because he gave a clinical outline. But I think in some ways we should differentiate between symptoms on the one hand and histological changes on the other. We do not know whether the histological changes link up with the clinical presentation. What is the relationship of the symptoms to cancer and what is the relationship of the histological changes to cancer? They are not nearly as progressive or as obvious as people seem to stress.

**Hughes**

I'm sure what you say is very important. Dr Junkermann too made the point that normal patients have abnormal histology and vice versa.

Dr Rasmussen, did you want to comment on what Dr Junkermann has said?

**Rasmussen**

Yes, I agree with Dr Junkermann, but it is not only a matter of the number of breast feedings or abrupt cessation of breast feeding. There is the factor also of heavy glandular structure and other factors relating to the dilatation and the development of cysts. I do not think our opinions are far apart.

**Leinster**

I'd like further clarification on this question of duct ectasia. It hasn't been my impression that patients who present with duct ectasia have had a previous history of cyclical pronounced mastalgia or anything else that we recognize as belonging to the fibrocystic disease/fibroadenosis spectrum. They have always seemed to me to be a separate group who present with a different problem and I've always treated them differently. But Dr Rasmussen implied that one progresses to the other.

**Hughes**

Yes, I think we have a real conflict in the way of terminology. Perhaps duct ectasia associated with discharge is different from duct ectasia associated with periductal inflammation. It may be that duct ectasia itself is a hormonal condition, but I don't think anyone has been able to prove that. Has anyone been able to show that there is an hormonal abnormality underlying duct ectasia? Mr Mansel, have you found a correlation in Texas?

**Mansel**

I don't think they are the same thing. Duct ectasia has never been shown to have any endocrinological correlation. It is a well-established histological condition and certainly in Cardiff we found the groups to be different, as I shall demonstrate later.

As Haagensen—the man who coined the term duct ectasia—has said, it is a well-defined condition which occurs throughout the age-ranges. It occurs in postmenopausal women and it is very common with dilated ducts and discharge at that age. I do not think there is any correlation.

**Hughes**

We're perhaps back in the province of coincidence and similarity. Dr Rasmussen's mention of cysts as a part of duct ectasia is an interesting concept. But you probably see more by doing duct injections than we see as surgeons.

**Shaikh**

Forgive me for being provocative, but what terms should we use when we write back to general practitioners? The patient has appeared with lumpiness. How do we describe it? Normally we use a variety of terms: fibroadenosis, fibrocystic disease, benign mammary dysplasia. In view of Dr Rasmussen's classification, I would like to suggest that we mix the terms so that instead of saying fibroadenosis with cystic changes, we say fibrocystadenosis. I'd like some views please.

**Hughes**

Could we have a general view on that? Is it possible to combine clinical and pathological descriptions? Or should we keep them separate and use the terms cystic mastopathy or hormonal mastopathy for the clinical group and keep the other terms for pathological changes.

**Gorins**

I would like to refer to apocrine changes which are very often observed in benign breast disease, with cells with a large eosinophilic pattern. I think these changes are important for prognosis and I would like some opinions about it.

**Hughes**

Apocrine changes are certainly very common. You say, Dr Gorins, that it is important for prognosis, but what do you think the significance is in relation to prognosis?

**Gorins**

I believe that when we see many metaplasic changes, it's a good thing for the patient.

**Hughes**

A good thing?

**Gorins**

Yes, that's my opinion.

**Hughes**

That's an interesting concept.

**Hermann**

As in most cases of benign breast disease we don't have mammography and in most cases we don't have histological studies, we in Bern think we should use mainly clinical terms, as suggested by Mr Preece, and not confound the issue with histological analysis which we in most cases do not have anyway.

**Hughes**

Thank you very much. Any other comments?

**Parbhoo**

Two of the authors have mentioned benign tumours as fibroadeno-mas, but this of course is still a controversial question and I wonder if any pathologists in the audience would like to comment on this?

Secondly, I would like to support Mr Lee in terms of the spectre of the risk of cancer. I think there are very few good studies with long-term follow-up of patients with, say, epitheliosis in terms of the actual incidence of cancer.

**Hughes**

First of all, are people talking about fibroadenoma tumour, meaning tumour as a lump or tumour as a neoplasm? Who used the term fibroadenoma? Or could we just accept that people don't regard fibroadenoma as being a tumour in the neoplastic sense, but rather a developmental abnormality?

Anyway, your point is well taken as is that of Mr Lee, that risk factors are still to be worked out. Although I think the work of Page and Haagensen is gradually giving us some data that will let us produce those figures sought by Dr Larue-Charlus.

# Session 2:
# Clinical and laboratory manifestations of breast disease

## CHAIRMAN'S INTRODUCTION

**L. E. HUGHES**

*University Department of Surgery,*
*Welsh National School of Medicine, Cardiff, Wales*

The papers in this second session are not as directly linked as those in the first session and so I propose to have a short period of discussion after each paper when any specific matter can be raised with the speaker.

*Benign Breast Disease, Edited by M. Baum, W. D. George, and L. E. Hughes, 1985: Royal Society of Medicine International Congress and Symposia series No. 76, published by The Royal Society of Medicine.*

# Benign breast disease—the cost to the service and the cost to the patient

## M. BAUM AND H. COOPER

*King's College Hospital Medical School,
London, England*

## Introduction

King's College Hospital serves a densely populated and deprived area of south-eastern London. A breast clinic was established there in January 1980 and, for the purpose of this paper, the impact of benign breast disease on this clinic has been reviewed for the first two years of its existence. Table 1 lists the numbers and percentages of each diagnostic sub-group seen at the clinic between January 1980 and December 1982. Although the single most common diagnosis was cancer (19 per cent), the large variety of benign breast pathology, together with those women with no apparent abnormality, accounted for the other 81 per cent. Just under half the patients who attended the clinic were discharged following clinical examination supplemented by mammography in selected cases. Patients presenting with simple cysts (13 per cent) were dealt with by single or multiple needle aspiration (see below),

*Table 1*
Attendances at King's College Hospital Breast Clinic (January 1980–December 1982)

| Diagnosis | No. | Percentage |
|---|---|---|
| Cancer | 244 | 19 |
| 'Lumpy breasts' | 224 | 17 |
| Normal breasts | 196 | 15 |
| Cysts | 167 | 13 |
| Mastalgia | 142 | 11 |
| Fibroadenoma | 116 | 9 |
| Duct ectasia complex | 63 | 6·5 |
| Epitheliosis } Sclerosing adenosis } | 53 | 4 |
| Duct papilloma | 19 | 1·5 |
| Miscellaneous | 48 | 5 |
| Total | 1292 | 100 |

*Benign Breast Disease, Edited by M. Baum, W. D. George, and L. E. Hughes, 1985: Royal Society of Medicine International Congress and Symposia series No. 76, published by The Royal Society of Medicine.*

19 per cent had discrete solid lumps or areas of mammographic suspicion which were subjected to open biopsy when no malignancy was found. This number is identical with the number of patients whose biopsy ultimately confirmed the presence of cancer. The proportion of one benign biopsy to one malignant biopsy compares favourably with other reported series from diagnostic clinics such as this (Abramson 1966; Hunt and Crass 1975), but a higher benign to malignant biopsy proportion might be expected from screening clinics (*British Medical Journal* 1976). It can be seen, therefore, that the overwhelming workload resulting from the establishment of a breast clinic is related to benign breast disease and yet the overwhelming research effort in this country is, of course, directed at cancer of the breast. Although benign breast disease is not life-threatening, nevertheless an attempt will be made to estimate its cost both from the patient's and from the health service's perspective, together with recommendations as to how these costs may be reduced.

## Cost of benign breast disease: patient's perspective

It is self-evident that the main problem from the patient's point of view is the intense anxiety associated with any symptom related to the breast, due to fear of cancer. This anxiety reaches a crescendo in the few days prior to the patient's attendance at the clinic. This has been estimated quantitatively in the past (Cheeseman *et al.* 1979) but can be easily demonstrated if a woman is asked about insomnia and the ingestion of alcohol or anxiolytics in the week preceding the first appointment at the clinic. If a biopsy is indicated, then a further intense period of anxiety builds up prior to the biopsy and while waiting for the result, so any attempts to reduce the biopsy rate must be applauded. Anxiety aside, serious cosmetic problems may result from repeated small biopsies, or removal of breast quadrants in the attempt to search for small mammographic abnormalities. A minority of patients presenting with mastalgia, in spite of being reassured that cancer is not present, will nevertheless continue to suffer from severe cyclical pain, which is a problem in its own right, and is dealt with in detail in subsequent papers at this symposium.

Finally, because of the intense publicity given to breast self-examination and early diagnosis of cancer, we are all beginning to see small numbers of women who are developing a neurosis resulting in increasing frequency of breast self-examination, with repeated attendances at the clinic for constant reassurance.

How then can we reduce the cost to the patient? It has taken many years to educate general practitioners that all discrete lumps in the breast must be viewed with suspicion and referred rapidly to the surgeon. It is our opinion that general practitioners have over-reacted towards extreme caution, and we think the time has come to re-educate them concerning which patients *not* to refer. This issue was discussed in detail in a recent publication (Baum and Preece 1983) and Table 2 lists the author's opinion on when general practitioners should, or should not, refer patients to the clinic. Once the general practitioner is convinced that a specialist opinion is required, then the waiting period must be reduced to a minimum and, if it is not possible for an open-house policy to be offered in a hospital, then at least the breast clinic should ensure that no woman has to wait for more than a week following the receipt of a referral letter. The patient having been seen in the clinic, if rapid reassurance cannot be provided following clinical examination and mammography, then histological diagnosis of the suspicious area must be expedited. Cyst aspiration or aspiration cytology should become more widely available and out-patient needle biopsy, with perhaps frozen section, may also reduce this period of uncertainty. Finally, and at the risk of being labelled an iconoclast, I think the time has come to

*Table 2*
*When referral is indicated*

| Refer | Do not refer |
| --- | --- |
| Discrete lump | Vague lumpiness (particularly if occurring just before menses) |
| Recent nipple retraction | Tender and/or enlarged costochondral junction |
| Circumferential nipple retraction | Long-standing nipple retraction |
| Serous/bloody nipple discharge | Linear nipple retraction white/cream/green nipple discharge |
| All ulcers | Superficial thromophlebitis |
| Eczema | Intertrigo |
| Mastalgia starting after 30 years of age (particularly if unilateral or non-cyclical) | Bilateral cyclical mastalgia under 30 years of age |

evaluate critically the whole subject of breast self-examination, asking the question: does breast self-examination save lives? (Baum 1982).

## Cost of benign breast disease—health service perspective

The establishment of a breast clinic involves enormous expenditure for the health service. The clinics themselves take up the time of medical, nursing and clerical staff. No breast clinic is complete without its mammography service and this involves capital outlay for the equipment and sessional payments for radiographers and radiologists. Inevitably, the establishment of such clinics increases the demand for beds and theatre time for in-patient biopsy.

Hospital costs could be reduced if the general practitioners were prepared to shoulder more of the responsibility for women presenting with breast symptoms. Also, out-patient biopsy or cytology would reduce the need for theatre time and bed occupancy, and a policy of repeatedly aspirating cysts might again reduce the biopsy rate.

It still surprises us that many clinicians, in many parts of the world, adhere to the obsolete notion that cyst aspiration is a hazardous procedure on the basis that an intracystic cancer might be missed and, also, that a solid tumour, if punctured, might disseminate the cancer. A number of recent publications have demonstrated the safety of this policy (Forrest *et al.* 1975; Hinton and Hughes 1981) and it is the intention to review critically our own policy with this in mind.

As with most other specialist centres in the United Kingdom, all women presenting with solitary cysts are treated by needle aspiration. On each reattendance, a new cyst appearing in a different part of the same breast, or in the contralateral breast, is aspirated. Biopsy is only indicated if any of the lumps turn out to be solid, if a residual lump is found at the site of aspiration at one month follow-up, if frank blood is found in the aspirate or if recurrent cysts occur at the same site as the original aspirated cysts. Finally, biopsy is of course indicated if mammography is reported as suspicious.

In the period under review, 130 cases were managed in this way (Table 3). There were 43 cases of cysts on the right side, 63 on the left and 24 bilateral cysts. Seventy-one per cent of patients were dealt with at a single aspiration, 20 per cent at two aspirations and the remaining 9 per cent required five or more aspirations, many of these patients continuing to return with new cysts at each visit. Of the total group, nearly 30 per cent were submitted to open biopsy, the outcome of which is shown in Table 4. Of these 38 patients, only three were subsequently shown to have cancer. One of these was a solid lump that had appeared during the follow-up of a woman with multiple cysts. The other two were intracystic cancers demonstrated by bloody fluid in the cyst aspirate. All nine of the suspicious mammograms were false positive and not one of the cases with a residual lump or recurrent cyst at the site of the first aspiration was positive. It can be concluded from this experience that a policy of cyst aspiration seems safe. Mammograms performed following cyst aspiration were not only unhelpful but positively misleading and, as with the experience of many other centres, solid lumps and bloody taps must be subjected to excision biopsy. There appear also to be two distinct cyst syndromes. One group of women presented with a solitary cyst which could be dealt with in one or two visits. The other group (about 10 per cent) go on and on continuing to form cysts. To date, an analysis of all demographic factors and drug history has failed to distinguish the type of women likely to develop one or other of these syndromes. Further research into the endocrine background of these two groups of patients is obviously indicated. Finally, as a result of this experience,

Table 3

Analysis of 130 cases*

|  | No. | Percentage |
|---|---|---|
| Single aspiration | 93 | 71 |
| Two aspirations | 26 | 20 |
| Five or more | 11 | 9 |
| Biopsy | 38 | 29 |

*Right breast, 43; left breast, 63; bilateral, 24 ($0.1 > P > 0.5$).

Table 4

Outcome of biopsies

| Indications | No. | Outcome | |
|---|---|---|---|
|  |  | Benign | Malignant |
| Solid lump | 1 | 0 | 1 |
| Bloody tap | 2 | 0 | 2 |
| Suspicious mammograms | 9 | 9 | 0 |
| Residual lump / Recurrent cyst | 26 | 26 | 0 |
| Total | 38 | 35 | 3 |

our policy for mammography has changed—all patients over the age of 30 referred to the clinic with breast symptoms have their mammogram performed before the clinical examination, as we suspect that a recently aspirated cyst may cause the radiologist difficulty in interpretation.

## Conclusions

Benign breast disease is a common problem which creates severe anxiety in many women and a heavy burden on an overstretched National Health Service. A policy of re-educating general practitioners when it is safe *not* to refer may reduce this problem. Cyst aspiration or needle aspiration cytology may also reduce the burden to both patient and health service. A critical evaluation of the cost effectiveness of mammography and breast self-examination is also urgently required.

Finally, I think it is important for all specialists to recognize their ignorance in this area. If nothing else this symposium has demonstrated that we cannot agree on the nomenclature of benign breast disease. We don't know its aetiology or natural history, therefore, it must be very difficult to evaluate its treatment! A great deal more research is needed, yet research costs money and most of the money available is directed into studies concerning breast cancer.

## References

Abramson, D. J. (1966). *Amer. J. Surg.,* **163**, 478.
Baum, M. (1982). *Brit. Med. J.,* **284**, 142.
Baum, M., and Preece, P. E. (1983). *Disorders of the breast: the practical GP guide.* Special Supplement to *Modern Medicine.*
*British Medical Journal* (1976). *Brit. Med. J.,* **ii**, 832.
Cheeseman, E., *et al.* (1979). *Clin. Oncol.* **5**, 194.
Forrest, A. P. M., *et al.* (1975). *Brit. Med. J.,* **3**, 30.
Hinton, C. P., and Hughes, R. G. (1981). *Brit. J. Surg.,* **68**, 45.
Hunt, T. K., and Crass, R. A. (1975). *Surg. Gynaecol. Obstet.,* **141**, 591.

## Discussion

**Powis**

Could I ask you Professor Baum why you don't send your biopsies for frozen section so the patient can have an answer when she wakes up?

**Baum**

You may well ask. I would like to do that.

**Powis**

I do, it works.

**Baum**

I know, you're lucky. But one needs collaboration.

**Mansel**

In discussing the re-aspirated cysts you didn't mention the role of the pneumocystogram. Isn't that a bit more useful here?

**Baum**

I went through a phase of doing pneumocystography and, in the ones that showed in intracyst cancer or an intracyst papilloma, they again had bloody fluid, all of them. I suppose inevitably we will one day miss the intracystic cancer, but pneumocystography is not an entirely benign procedure. I have seen one abscess develop as a result of pneumocystography.

**Lee**

An excellent paper. There is just one thing I'd like to question and that is the idea of educating general practitioners not to send patients. We, as you know, are a district hospital and we do not get specialized referral from other places. In a study carried out in Daventry and mirrored by other general practitioner studies, it was found that only about 20 per cent of the patients who present to the GP with breast symptoms get referred to hospital. Furthermore, three-quarters of our cancer patients present with very large nodes and 6 per cent have very large and ulcerated cancers. When we analysed the ones with the nodes, we found that something like 30 per cent of them had been seen by a GP within the year before they came to the hospital with a cancer. My suggestion is that whilst education is absolutely essential it may not be just a matter of educating GPs not to send, but rather of educating them in the examination of their patients so that the patients they do not send are only the ones that you put in the 'Do not send' category.

**Baum**

Thank you Mr Lee, your point is well taken. Education is certainly the answer to the question of whether or not the GP should refer.

**Hughes**

Are you happy Mr Lee with the criteria that Professor Baum put up for referral?

**Lee**

I think there are a number of different arguments but, in general, yes.

**Kumar**

Referring to your figures of 71 per cent single aspiration, 20 per cent double aspiration and 9 per cent repeated aspiration in cyst disease, how long was the follow-up? We certainly have seen patients who return four or five years after the first or second aspiration.

**Baum**

That's a good point because I have been at King's for only three-and-a-half years, so that is the maximum follow-up I have. But we do have an open-door policy and on leaving the clinic after two visits, if the cyst hasn't recurred at three months, the patient is given (I'm embarrassed to say!) a leaflet on self-examination and instructed to come back if the cyst should recur. It's likely that we've missed one or two recurrences but nevertheless there does seem to be a clear pattern of two cyst-type syndromes.

**Hinton**

I can't let the comments on breast self-examination go entirely unanswered. In Nottingham we are part of the DHSS study into breast-screening involved in our programme of breast self-examination, and we've educated some 35 000 women in the technique. Whether or not it saves lives is a question that remains to be answered, but the indications are that it probably does in that the tumours are smaller and there is less node involvement than we were experiencing before. The question of neurosis we found to be a minimal problem, to our surprise. There are a few women who continually come back to the self-referral centres with what we consider to be normal breasts, perhaps with diffuse lumpiness, but it's been a very small problem in this programme.

**Baum**

I think that's a very important point. The Department of Health in Britain is funding this serious project to evaluate breast self-examination and what you've just described would certainly prolong the period of observation of patients with cancer without, however, necessarily saving their lives.

**Morrison**

I agree with you that thermography has little value in breast cysts. A technique that is widely used when aspirating breast cysts that I don't think you mentioned is that of doing cytology on the fluid, and that technique is of no value either. We did it for many years and when we reviewed the results we found it to be useless in terms of cost-effectiveness.

**Hughes**

Just before we finish, could I ask Dr Rasmussen if he would like to comment on that question of two populations of cysts, because radiologists see a lot of cysts with duct injection, particularly on the Continent?

**Rasmussen**

Yes. I agree with nearly all that Professor Baum has said and I have the same impression, that there are cysts, mostly in very heavy glandular tissue, which are 'once-only' cysts, that is they will never recur, and with such cysts no secretion can be expressed from the nipples. And then there is the other type, the cysts that may have been recurring for 30 years, until the patient reaches the mid-menopause, when there will be no more of them.

**Hughes**

Obviously there is still a lot to be learned about cysts. I think that to reduce the 19 per cent biopsy figure we need more research, more of the hormonal background, the pathogenesis, and perhaps the hormonal manipulation of these patients, to get rid of the nodularities that lead to these unnecessary biopsies.

# Classification of mastalgia—the Cardiff system

## R. E, MANSEL*

*Department of Medicine, Division of Oncology,
The University of Texas, Houston, Texas, USA*

I want to talk today about an empirical classification of benign breast disease which we designed some years ago in the Cardiff Breast Clinic. This system is simple to use and seems to have some interesting correlations with endocrinology rather than pathology.

The confusion that surrounds the clinicopathological descriptions of benign breast disease is well illustrated in a review which appeared recently in the *New England Journal of Medicine* (1982). Under the heading 'Fibrocystic "disease" of the breast—a nondisease?' the authors asked,

> 'Is fibrocystic disease a distinct entity? Is it a diagnosis that can be made clinically or histologically? Does this designation imply an increased risk of breast cancer? Should we attempt to treat it?'

The authors went on critically to review the literature that had appeared on the subject since 1964 and came to the conclusion that there is no such disease. They reached this conclusion because it became clear that the histology of benign breast disease has virtually no correlation with the clinical presentations.

It was for this very reason that in 1973 we designed a symptomatic classification which has now been in use for the last 10 years.

The classification is based on a simple recording of the relationship of the symptoms of pain and the signs of nodularity with the phases of the menstrual cycle. A chart (Fig. 1) is given to each patient referred to the Breast Pain Clinic after a history of all the relevant menstrual and reproductive factors has been taken and after clinical examination and mammography to exclude breast cancer. The patient is asked to use the chart to record the days when pain has been experienced, the degree of the pain and the days of menstruation.

Figure 2 is a typical chart of a 'normal' patient, showing a few days of mild pain before each menstrual period. It has been estimated that almost 50 per cent of women have a pattern of this kind; such women should by no means be considered to be 'diseased'.

A completely different type of patient record is illustrated in Fig. 3. The patient has a pattern of prolonged, severe pain, present for about half the cycle and clearly related

*Previous appointment: Senior Lecturer, Hon. Consultant Surgeon, University Hospital of Cardiff, Wales.

Benign Breast Disease, *Edited by M. Baum, W. D. George, and L. E. Hughes, 1985: Royal Society of Medicine International Congress and Symposia series No. 76, published by The Royal Society of Medicine.*

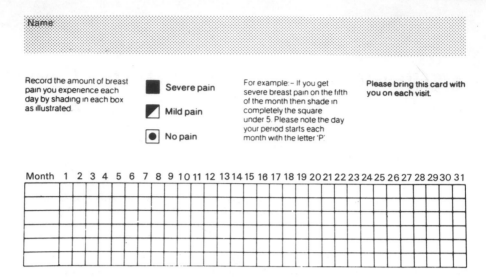

Fig. 1. Daily breast pain chart.

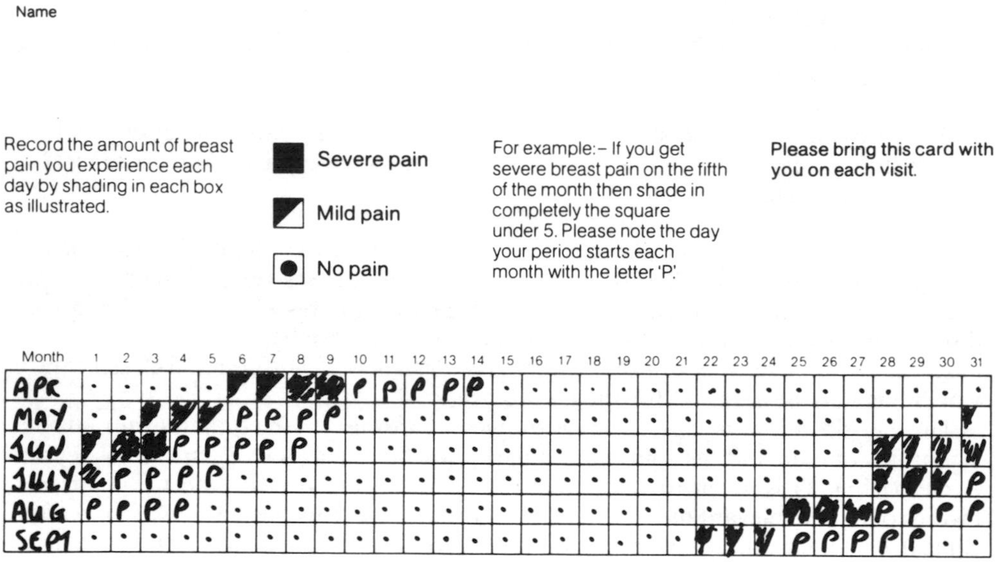

Fig. 2. Daily breast pain chart—'normal' patient.

to it. This is the cyclical type and the commonest, making up some 40 per cent of the total.

Figure 4 illustrates the clinical features of the cyclical pattern. The pain is cyclical, prolonged and generally localized to the upper outer quadrants of the breasts, although it has a diffuse quality. The pain is often bilateral although it occurs slightly more frequently in the left breast. Nodularity is common. The descriptive terms 'heaviness and tenderness' are commonly used by patients. The average age is about 34 years.

Name

Record the amount of breast pain you experience each day by shading in each box as illustrated.

Severe pain

Mild pain

No pain

For example:– If you get severe breast pain on the fifth of the month then shade in completely the square under 5. Please note the day your period starts each month with the letter 'P'.

**Please bring this card with you on each visit.**

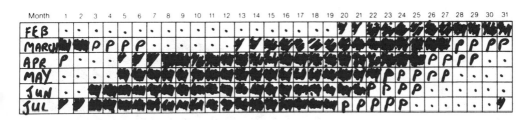

Fig. 3. Daily breast pain chart—cyclical pattern.

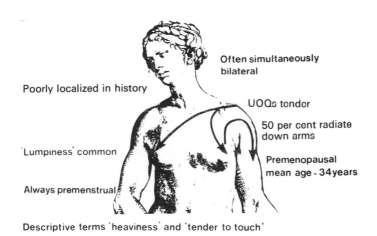

Often simultaneously bilateral

Poorly localized in history

UOQs tender

50 per cent radiate down arms

'Lumpiness' common

Premenopausal mean age - 34 years

Always premenstrual

Descriptive terms 'heaviness' and 'tender to touch'

Fig. 4. Cyclical pattern—clinical features.

The non-cyclical pattern is illustrated by the chart shown in Fig. 5. This is the second largest group seen. There is no obvious relationship with the menstrual cycle, although the pain is not continuous. The degree of pain in these patients appears to be less than in the cyclical group.

The clinical features of the non-cyclical group are illustrated in Fig. 6. Patients are older, with a mean age of 43, and they include both pre- and postmenopausal women. The pain is well localized in the breast, often on one side only. Frequently there is little or no nodularity around the site of the pain. The descriptive words used are 'drawing' and 'burning'. Other workers have referred to a sharp, tingling sensation when these localized pains are palpated and have used the term 'trigger-spot' pain to describe the phenomenon. Originally, we associated this pattern with duct ectasia, but

Name

Record the amount of breast pain you experience each day by shading in each box as illustrated.

 Severe pain

Mild pain

No pain

For example:- If you get severe breast pain on the fifth of the month then shade in completely the square under 5. Please note the day your period starts each month with the letter 'P'.

Please bring this card with you on each visit.

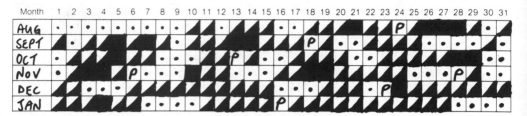

*Fig. 5. Daily breast pain chart—non-cyclical pattern.*

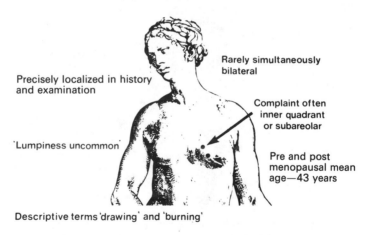

Rarely simultaneously bilateral

Precisely localized in history and examination

Complaint often inner quadrant or subareolar

'Lumpiness uncommon'

Pre and post menopausal mean age—43 years

Descriptive terms 'drawing' and 'burning'

*Fig. 6. Non-cyclical pattern—clinical features.*

since we have been unable to find a relationship with the pathology of duct ectasia, we now use the term 'non-cyclical'.

The third largest group is that of Tietze's disease—the painful costo-chondral syndrome (Fig. 7). This, of course, is not true breast pain. It is a condition well known to physicians and surgeons alike and can be differentiated from the pain occurring in the non-cyclical group by the presence of tender costal cartilages. The condition is self-limiting and usually requires only reassurance, although there have been reports of good results from injections of local anaesthetic around the painful cartilages.

The main patterns of mastalgia seen in the Cardiff clinic in the first five years are shown in Table 1. The cyclical pronounced group was the commonest, followed by the non-cyclical group (described as 'duct ectasia' in the table) and then the fairly

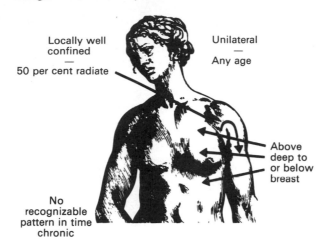

Locally well
confined
—
50 per cent radiate

Unilateral
—
Any age

Above
deep to
or below
breast

No
recognizable
pattern in time
chronic

*Fig. 7. Tietze disease—clinical features.*

*Table 1*
*Patterns of mastalgia (Cardiff Breast Clinic, first 5 years)*

| Classification | No. patients |
|---|---|
| Cyclical pronounced | 93 |
| Duct ectasia | 62 |
| Tietze syndrome | 25 |
| *Trauma* | *19* |
| Sclerosing adenosis | 11 |
| Cancer | 1 |
| Miscellaneous | 21 |
| Total | 232 |

common Tietze's syndrome group. Post-trauma cases were less frequent, although we had a number of patients who had had a complicated biopsy, usually a haematoma following a benign biopsy, which reinforces the point made by Professor Baum earlier in this symposium about the cost to the patient of biopsy. Less frequent still was sclerosing adenosis and non-breast causes such as cervical root syndrome and even gall stones. Only a single cancer case appears in the table because patients with obvious or early cancer were referred to a breast clinic and so were removed from this study. Here it is worth noting that when Paul Preece reviewed the relationship between mastalgia and cancer in 240 patients with operable cancer, he found that 7 per cent presented with pain only; a further 8 per cent presented with pain and lump together. It is therefore clearly important always to be aware that cancer can be present when there is pain.

We have now examined and classified some 800 women in detail and the system of classification remains useful. It might be thought that this system is too simple to work satisfactorily; however, three different pieces of evidence have recently emerged from work conducted at the Cardiff clinic which have reinforced the conviction that the system will continue to prove useful.

The first piece of evidence emerged from a trial of bromocriptine that we carried out on two groups of breast pain patients in which the effects of treatment on heaviness, tenderness and sex-life problems were assessed. Compared with the pre-trial situation and the effects of placebo, there was a positive response to bromocriptine in patients in the cyclical pain group (Fig. 8). However, patients in the non-cyclical group did not respond to the antihormonal agent (Fig. 9). Thus, the separation of the two groups on symptomatic grounds seems to predict the results of therapy.

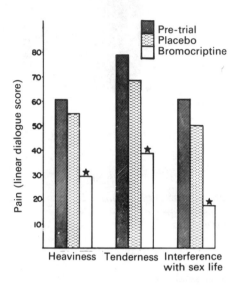

Fig. 8. Cyclical pain group: bromocriptine trial. Asterisk indicates $P < 0.05$ in Wilcoxon's signed rank test.

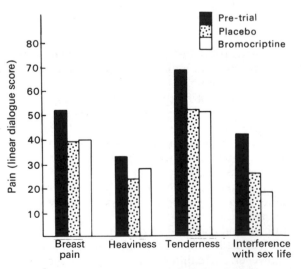

Fig. 9. Non-cyclical group: bromocriptine trial. No significant differences between placebo and bromocriptine treatment.

The second piece of evidence came from a study of pituitary function, by means of a TRH/domperidone stimulation test, in benign breast disease patients before therapy. Serum prolactin levels after the administration of 200 µg TRH i.v. were very much higher in the cyclical mastalgia patients than in either non-cyclical patients or normal controls (Fig. 10). The difference was significant not only at the peak point but 60 min later. Hence, the cyclical group, selected on a simple symptom basis, responded differently to a test of hormonal activity.

Finally, in a study in which serum unsaturated fatty acid precursors of prostaglandin production were measured, different baseline levels of the fatty acid metabolites of linoleic acid were found in the two benign breast disease groups compared with normals, and the pattern in cyclical patients was significantly different from that seen in non-cyclical patients. This study is continuing at the present time and promises to yield interesting results.

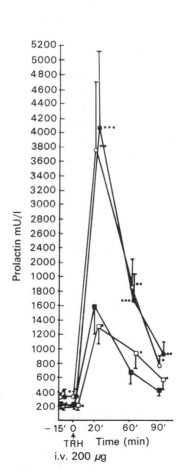

Fig. 10. Serum prolactin after TRH. ●——●, nodular breast disease (n=10); ○——○, cyclical mastalgia (n=17); ■——■, control (n=11); □——□, non-cyclical mastalgia (n=7). All points are means ±S.E. *P=n.s.; **P<0.05; ***P<0.02.

# Discussion

**Gorins**

I would like to ask Mr Mansel his views on whether or not breast pain can have its origin in the cervical spine. Secondly, whether he thinks breast pain can occur without organic cause at all, that is, pain which has a psychological origin. I have a comment, too, on the TRH test he discussed; when I give my paper shortly, I shall present some results which are not in perfect accord with the results he showed.

**Mansel**

Yes, it's a very common occurrence to get pain radiating from the cervical spine. Everyone looking at cases of mastalgia has seen many instances where the pain has been caused by cervical spondylosis. In the groups I presented, such cases were excluded. Only cases of what we call true breast pain were included. Other types of pain, including pain arising from angina and gall stones, as I mentioned, appeared in the table I showed you under the 'Miscellaneous' heading.

As far as pain of psychological origin is concerned, we looked at this and published a paper on the subject in the *British Medical Journal*. We looked at psychoneuroses in such patients and examined psychoneurotic profiles, but we found it difficult to determine if the psychology led to the pain or if the pain was more complained of because of the psychology. However, we did find that the mastalgia group of patients was no different from a surgical outpatients group. Some patients did require psychiatric treatment and we referred these patients for therapy of this kind.

**Hughes**

What you're saying is that mastalgia patients are no more neurotic than any other surgical patients?

**Mansel**

That's right, that was our finding.

**Gumpert**

Can I ask about your 240 operable cancers, 7 per cent of which presented with pain? This is obviously a fairly disturbing statistic. Can you give us more details of these patients? What sort of pain did they have? Did they respond to bromocriptine? Was their pain cyclical or non-cyclical?

**Mansel**

These patients were not treated for mastalgia; they were analysed retrospectively. Mr Paul Preece did the analysis, so perhaps he can comment on whether the character of the pain had any predictive value.

**Preece**

The situation is even more disturbing when one looks at that point, because these patients had all types of pain. There was nothing in the adjectives they used to describe the pain they had which might give one a clue. Both Mr Mansel and I can call vividly to mind that three patients in this group whose cancer was not declared for quite a long time and about whom, of course, we had very red faces afterwards. I can't give you anything which would help you suspect cancer, except for one point which we specified, and that is that a new unilateral pain after the age of 30 should be taken very seriously.

**Gumpert**

Has this changed your attitude in any way, Mr Preece? Do you, for example, refer patients for mammography more readily than you otherwise would?

**Preece**

I think the honest answer to that is probably, yes. I have been fortunate to have been working in a specialized clinic for quite some time and we have tended to do mammography in that setting to enable us to get research information. But I think if I were practising outside that setting, I would probably be using mammography rather more because of this.

**Hughes**

Would you say that if you had localized persistent pain, you would repeat a mammogram in a year?

**Preece**

Yes. In these three particularly difficult cases, mammography was very helpful. There is one interesting slant, if I may mention it whilst we're on the subject, because it is important in this area. A high proportion of these tumours have turned out ultimately to have lobular histology and it is well known that these do not declare themselves well on mammograms at an early phase and also that they are very difficult on frozen section.

**Hughes**

And have a good prognosis in general?

**Preece**

Yes, a reasonable prognosis.

# The contribution of infra-red thermography to the diagnosis of benign breast disease

## A. GORINS, R. THIERREE AND P. SAUVAL

*University of Paris VIIIᵉ, Hôpital St Louis, Paris, France*

Thermography of the breast offers an interesting method of investigating breast disease. Certainly its reliability in the diagnosis of cancer has been challenged, but this is something we do not wish to discuss here.

We believe that thermography is a useful procedure for evaluating the condition of the mammary gland, two criteria being essentially considered—overall temperature and vascularization.

In this paper, we propose to deal only with infra-red thermography and to demonstrate first those thermographic appearances considered to be normal, however with certain physiological variations; second, several cases of breast cancer; and finally, the thermographic presentation of benign breast disease.

**Figures 1–15 in this paper are to be found in the colour section at the end of the symposia.**

*Benign Breast Disease, Edited by M. Baum, W. D. George, and L. E. Hughes, 1985: Royal Society of Medicine International Congress and Symposia series No. 76, published by The Royal Society of Medicine.*

# Discussion

### Lloyd-Williams

Professor Gorins is quite right when he says that thermography has had a very bad press. Perhaps too bad. We should beware of throwing the baby out with the bath water. Thermography is a physiological tool. It does reflect the vasculature and hormone activity of the breast. A woman can be recognized by her mammary thermal profile and a change in this is significant. Ovulation can be determined by taking serial thermographic pictures of the breasts. A consistently positive thermogram carries a high risk of developing breast cancer and the degree of asymmetry gives a fairly accurate assessment of prognosis.

Inflammatory carcinoma of the breast is said to have an incidence of 4 per cent. If one measures the temperature difference and accepts all cases over 3 °C, an incidence of 12 per cent is produced. These cases have a uniformly bad prognosis: 80 per cent are dead at two-and-a-half years and 100 per cent at five years with conventional therapy, exactly the same sort of prognosis as cases diagnosed clinically. I think we should avoid an attitude of 'tried it once and didn't like it'. The equipment is now very reliable, although expensive. The rheumatologists are finding thermography a valuable tool in the measurement of drug effects and we may find that we, too, have a use for it, in unravelling benign breast disease and the effects of hormones upon it.

### Hughes

Professor Gorins, is thermography a first-line investigation in your clinic or do you do mammography first?

### Gorins

Yes, we do mammography first. Thermography is an investigative procedure which has a place beside other investigative methods, for example mammography and echography; we never interpret thermograms in isolation. Never.

# Hormonal profile of benign breast disease and premenstrual mastodynia

## A. GORINS, R. THIERREE AND P. SAUVAL

*University of Paris VIII\u1d49, Hôpital St Louis,
Paris, France*

## Patients and methods

This study was carried out on 171 patients. Of these, 82 were cases of major benign breast disease, and it is worth noting that it is not unusual for even major benign breast disease not to be accompanied by acute painful episodes in the menstrual period. Of the remainder, 71 were cases of benign breast disease associated with mastodynia with premenstrual recrudescence, the intensity and/or duration of which was definitely pathological, and 18 cases of premenstrual mastodynia without obvious associated benign breast disease. The classification of these 171 cases merits careful differentiation since some cases of benign breast disease may be accompanied by mastodynia on some occasions but not on others.

We carried out plasma assays of oestradiol ($E_2$), progesterone (PG), testosterone (T) and prolactin (PRL), and in some cases a TRH-stimulation test was also performed. Hormonal assays by a radioimmunological technique were carried out in the second half of the cycle, on average between the fourth and eighth day after ovulation, based on the displacement of the BBT curve.

All these patients presented with ovulatory cycles. No patient was taking oral contraceptives and none was receiving long-term hormone therapy.

Some patients received several assays every two days during the luteal phase, although the majority of the women who were followed up as out-patients had only one assay.

## Results

The mean age of the patients with major benign breast disease but without mastodynia was 38 years, with a range of 21–50 years (Fig. 1). Figure 2 shows that the oestradiol values as assayed fell within normal physiological limits. Progesterone values also fell within normal limits (Fig. 3). From Fig. 4, it will be seen that the base values for prolactin almost always fell within normal limits, that is below 15 ng/ml, and that after TRH stimulation an increased response was seen in only one of the eight tests performed.

*Benign Breast Disease, Edited by M. Baum, W. D. George, and L. E. Hughes, 1985: Royal Society of Medicine International Congress and Symposia series No. 76, published by The Royal Society of Medicine.*

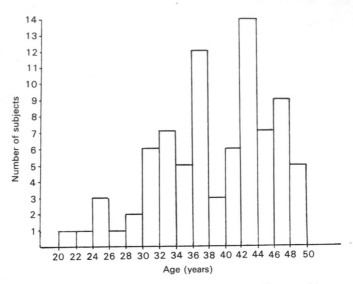

Fig. 1. *Age distribution of 82 patients with benign breast disease. Mean age 38 years; range 21–50 years.*

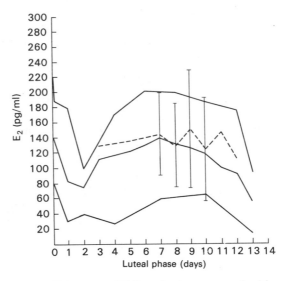

Fig. 2. *Luteal phase oestradiol assays: BBD patients compared with controls. ——, usual (control) values; – – –, observed values (patients).*

In the majority of cases, the progesterone/oestradiol ratio ($PG/E_2$) fell within the normal limits of 0·8 and 1·2 (Fig. 5). There appeared to be no differences in the distribution of results either side of the normal range.

Overall, hypoprogesteronaemia was found in 14 per cent of patients in this group and hyperprogesteronaemia in 5 per cent; hypo-oestrogenaemia was found in 14 per cent and hyperoestrogenaemia in 21 per cent.

In the group of patients with major benign breast disease who had severe premenstrual mastodynia, the age range was 19–52 years, with a mean of 37 years

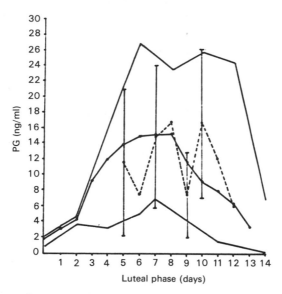

Fig. 3. Luteal phase plasma progesterone levels (PG): BBD patients compared with controls. ———, usual (control) values; – – –, observed values (patients).

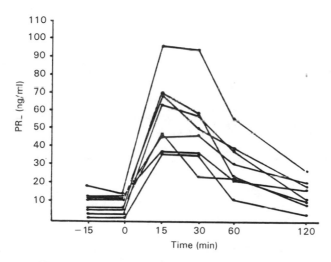

Fig. 4. Prolactin (PRL) assays—BBD patients.

(Fig. 6). Except for two assays out of nine (the significance of which is subject to some reservation because of the small number of assays), oestradiol values fell within physiological limits (Fig. 7). Figure 8 gives the values for the progesterone assays, again falling with normal limits. Base values for prolactin fell mostly within normal limits; after TRH stimulation, two increased responses were seen out of the seven tests carried out (Fig. 9).

In the majority of cases, the progesterone/oestradiol ratio ($PG/E_2$) fell within normal limits and there appeared to be no differences in the distribution of the results either side of the values regarded as normal (Fig. 10).

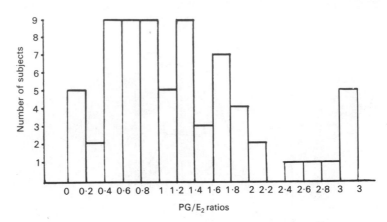

Fig. 5. PG/E₂ ratios in patients with benign breast disease.

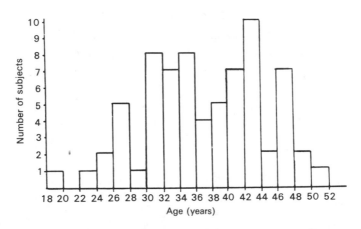

Fig. 6. Age distribution of patients with benign breast disease and premenstrual mastodynia. Mean age 37 years; range 19–52 years.

Overall, hypoprogesteronaemia was found in 7 per cent of patients in this group and hyperprogesteronaemia in 6 per cent; hypo-oestrogenaemia was found in 4 per cent and hyperoestrogenaemia in 22 per cent.

In the final group of patients—those with isolated premenstrual mastodynia—the age range was 21–47 years with a mean of 37 years (Fig. 11). Two out of 17 patients in this group assayed for oestradiol had values above normal limits (11 per cent) and five out of 18 patients (28 per cent) had progesterone values below normal limits.

In the 14 prolactin assays, no base levels were found to be abnormal; in the five TRH-stimulation tests carried out, one single, strong response was observed (Fig. 12).

## Comments and conclusions

On the evidence of this study, it appears that hormonal imbalance is not a constant feature of benign breast disease and/or mastodynia. Oestrogen luteal imbalance with absolute excess of $E_2$ or insufficient levels of PG or an abnormal PG/$E_2$ ratio is likely to be found in only a minority of such patients.

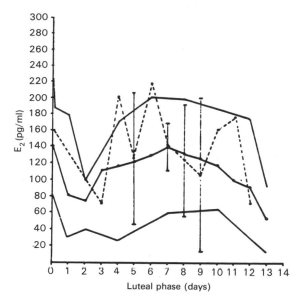

Fig. 7. Luteal phase oestradiol levels: patients with BBD and premenstrual mastodynia compared with controls. ——, usual (control) values; – – –, observed values (patients).

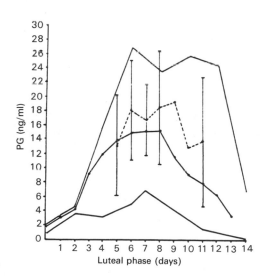

Fig. 8. Luteal phase progesterone values: patients with BBD and premenstrual mastodynia compared with controls. ——, usual (control) values; – – –, observed values (patients).

It would appear that fewer than one woman in four presents with a basal anomaly of the three major mammary trophic hormones—$E_2$, PG, PRL. Furthermore, the hypophyseal responses of PRL to TRH stimulation frequently remain within accepted physiological limits (excessive responses observed being interpreted in the context of the hormonal situation of the post-ovulatory phase of the menstrual cycle).

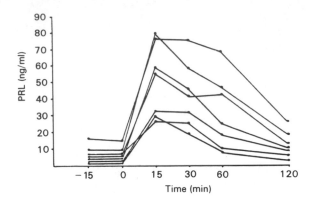

Fig. 9. *Dynamic assay of prolactin levels: patients with BBD and premenstrual mastodynia.*

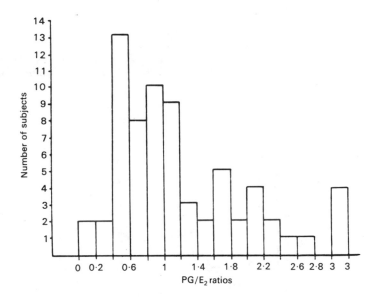

Fig. 10. *PG/E₂ ratios: patients with BBD and premenstrual mastodynia.*

## Summary

The results of the plasma assays conducted in this study, considered in isolation from such factors as hormone receptors and/or the local receptivity of the mammary glands, confirm the absence of a constant oestrogen luteal imbalance and of dysprolactinaemia in benign breast disease and/or premenstrual mastodynia.

## Discussion

[Discussion of this paper is combined with that of the following paper: see pp. 57–60.]

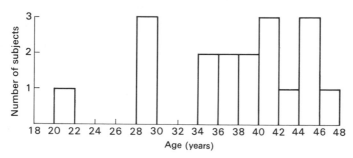

Fig. 11. Age distribution of patients with premenstrual mastodynia.

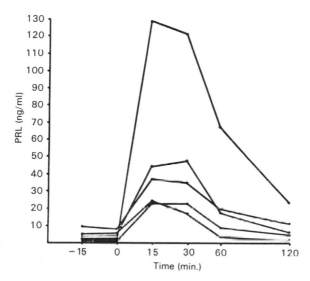

Fig. 12. Dynamic assay of prolactin levels: patients with premenstrual mastodynia.

# Luteal phase function and benign breast disease

## P. V. WALSH, K. MORRIS, I. W. McDICKEN, G. H. WHITEHOUSE AND W. D. GEORGE

*University Departments of Surgery, Pathology and Radiodiagnosis, and Department of Chemical Pathology, Royal Liverpool Hospital, Liverpool, England*

The aetiology of benign breast disease is unknown, but it does seem reasonable to consider that at least some forms may have an endocrine basis, particularly cyclical mastodynia, where the symptoms of pain and swelling seem to coincide so well with the luteal phase.

To digress for a moment from benign disease, the 'inadequate luteal phase hypothesis' was proposed as a possible explanation for the cause of at least a proportion of cases of breast cancer, the deficient production of progesterone leaving the oestrogens unopposed, thus perhaps inducing or enhancing breast cancer risk.

In a sense, there was some support for this hypothesis from the work of Mauvais-Jarvis *et al.* (1980), who found a subnormal concentration of progesterone in women with various types of benign breast disease (Fig. 1). These subnormal concentrations were found in the presence of normal concentrations of oestradiol, or even with increased oestradiol concentrations in women with fibroadenoma.

Earlier workers (England *et al.* 1975), however, had demonstrated a normal progesterone profile in women with benign disease, but they also found a tendency towards a higher concentration of oestradiol during the latter part of the luteal phase in these patients. These workers and others (Cole *et al.* 1977) also reported an increased concentration of prolactin in relation to some forms of benign disease, particularly painful breast disease.

We undertook our work in the light of this apparent controversy. The aim of our study was to investigate the concentrations of progesterone, oestradiol and prolactin during the luteal phase of the menstrual cycle in women with cyclical mastodynia and in patients with biopsied benign breast disease.

## Methods

Multiple blood samples were obtained from women in three groups during the luteal phase of the menstrual cycle. Samples were taken in the evening and each was dated according to the number of days that elapsed before the next menstrual period.

*Benign Breast Disease, Edited by M. Baum, W. D. George, and L. E. Hughes, 1985: Royal Society of Medicine International Congress and Symposia series No. 76, published by The Royal Society of Medicine.*

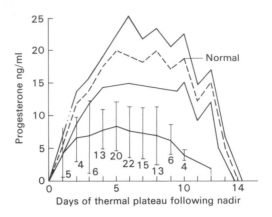

Fig. 1. *Concentration of progesterone in women with various types of breast disease (109 patients with mastopathy; values are means±S.E.M.).*

Group C consisted of 33 patients with persistent, severe and disabling cyclical breast pain. In the second group (group B), there were 14 normal women acting as controls. These women had no breast symptoms, no history of breast disease, no family history of breast cancer and no history of involuntary infertility. On both clinical and radiological examination, their breasts were normal. The third group (group D) was of 54 women who had undergone breast biopsy for a benign condition within the previous two years.

The histology slides of each of the biopsied women were reviewed by a single pathologist (I.W.M.) and the appearances classified according to the presence or absence of epithelial proliferation. Hormone concentrations were determined by radioimmunoassay.

## Results

Figure 2 shows the progesterone profiles of patients with severe cyclical mastodynia (group C) compared with those of the normal (group B) women. No evidence of progesterone deficiency was found in the breast pain patients.

Similarly, no evidence of progesterone deficiency was found in patients biopsied for benign breast disease (group D) when their progesterone profiles were compared with those of the control group (Fig. 3). Even when the biopsied women were separated according to whether their biopsies did or did not show epitheliosis, there was no evidence to indicate progesterone deficiency in women who might be considered to be at high risk (Fig. 4).

Figure 5 shows the serum oestradiol profiles of patients with cyclical breast pain compared with normal women. Whereas oestradiol levels in normal women appeared to fall towards the latter part of the luteal phase, in the cyclical breast pain patients, the levels tended to remain high. This difference just reached statistical significance ($P < 0.05$). In Fig. 6, the profiles of women who have been biopsied are compared with those of the normal women. Again, there was a tendency towards a higher concentration of oestradiol during the latter part of the luteal phase in the biopsied women, and this again reached statistical significance ($P < 0.01$).

Serum prolactin profiles for cyclical pain patients and normal controls are shown in Fig. 7. As with oestradiol, there was a tendency for prolactin concentrations to be

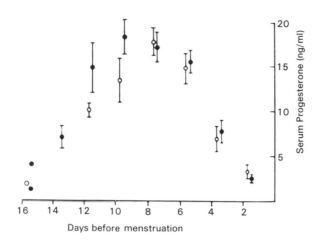

Fig. 2. Progesterone profiles of patients with cyclical mastodynia (●, *group C) compared with normal controls (○, group B).*

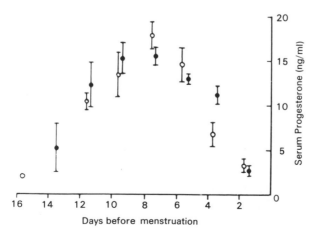

*Fig. 3. Progesterone profiles of biopsied patients (●, group D, n=54) compared with normal controls (○, group B).*

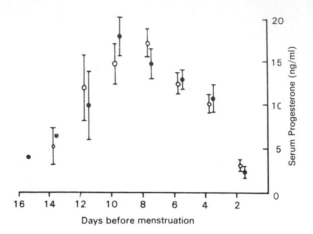

Fig. 4. Progesterone levels with (●) and without (○) epitheliosis.

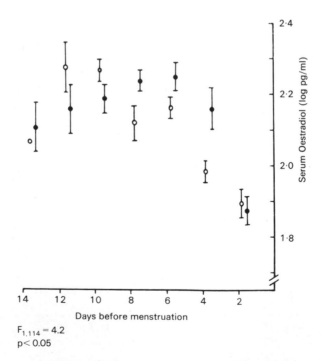

$F_{1, 114} = 4.2$
$p < 0.05$

Fig. 5. Oestradiol profiles of patients with cyclical mastodynia (●, group C) compared with normal controls (○, group B) ($F_{1, 114} = 4.3$; $P < 0.05$).

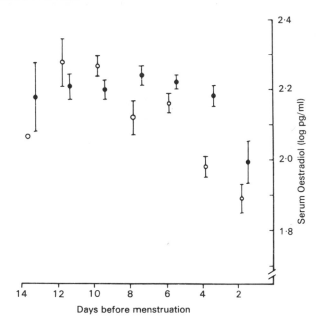

Fig. 6. *Oestradiol profiles of biopsied patients (●, group D, n=54) compared with normal controls (○, group B).*

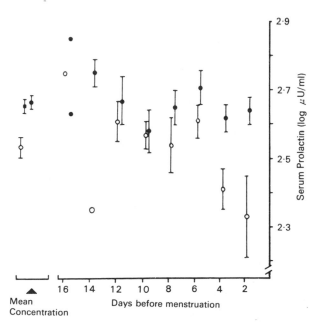

Fig. 7. *Prolactin profiles of patients with cyclical mastodynia (●, group C) compared with normal controls (○, group B).*

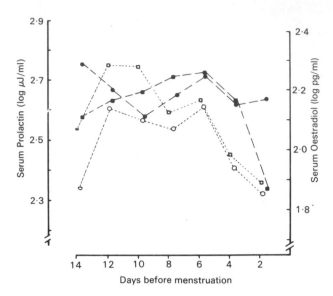

Fig. 8. *Mean oestradiol and prolactin profiles in patients with cyclical mastodynia (group C) compared with normal controls (group B).* ●−−−●, *prolactin, group C;* ○−−−○, *prolactin, group B;* ■−−−■, *oestradiol, group C;* □−−−□, *oestradiol, group B.*

higher during the latter part of the luteal phase of cyclical pain patients compared with the control women, whose prolactin levels fall. The much higher mean concentration for the cyclical pain patients is statistically significant ($P < 0.01$).

The results in respect of the two hormones, oestradiol and prolactin, show a parallel trend, demonstrated in Fig. 8.

Although, in the patients who had been biopsied, the prolactin concentrations again tended to remain high during the latter part of the luteal phase compared with normal controls (Fig. 9), there was no significant difference between the mean concentrations in the two groups.

As with progesterone, the oestrogen and prolactin profiles of the biopsied women showed no variation with histological appearance.

In this study, then, we found no evidence of progesterone deficiency in women with benign breast disease. On the other hand, and as has been previously reported, we did find an increased concentration of oestradiol during the latter part of the luteal phase and the concentration of prolactin, known to be influenced by oestrogens, appeared to reflect the oestradiol abnormality, particularly in respect of painful disease.

## Conclusions

These results may indicate an abnormality of oestrogen production or metabolism in women with benign breast disease, as previously reported by England *et al.* (1974) and this may be reflected in an abnormal measurable concentration of prolactin.

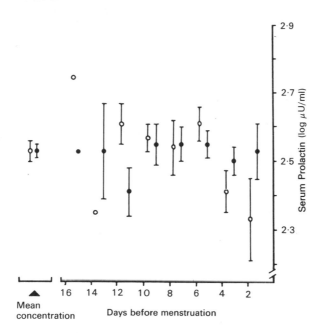

**Fig. 9.** *Prolactin levels of biopsied patients (●, group D, n=54) compared with normal controls (○, group B).*

# References

Cole, E. M., *et al.* (1977). *Brit. J. Cancer,* **13**, 597–603.
England, P. C., *et al.* (1974). *Brit. J. Cancer,* **30**, 517–76.
England, P. C., *et al.* (1975). *Brit. J. Surg.,* **62**, 806–9.
Mauvais-Jarvis, P., *et al.* (1980). In *Commentaries on research in breast disease* (eds R. D. Bulbisola and D. J. Taylor), Vol. 1, pp. 22–59. Allan R. Liss, New York.

# Discussion

[This discussion incorporates discussion of the paper by Gorins *et al.* on pp. 43–49.]

### Hughes

It's quite obvious that the endocrine background to benign breast disease is no clearer than is the terminology and I think that it is very important to assess the present situation.

### Kumar

I would like to make a brief comment on Professor Gorin's paper. I'm glad he brought up the point that out of seven patients with mastodynia, there were two who had abnormal TRH tests. In the data earlier presented by Mr Mansel, it was very clearly shown that in about half the number of patients the TRH test was not abnormal, while the other half did have very high abnormal rates. That is always the case with the TRH test: there are explosive responses and there are responses of the same order as those seen in normal women. That is why we looked into the other limb of prolactin secretion, the regulation of prolactin secretion, which is more important. Inhibiting dopamine by using domperidone, a dopamine antagonist somewhat like metoclopramide, we found that the prolactin abnormality was even more consistent. However, it is very important that these tests are carried out under strict statistical control, because in the data collected there are large differences between the basal prolactin levels and the stimulated prolactin levels.

**Hughes**

Professor Gorins, do you have any experience of the domperidone test?

**Gorins**

No, we do not, but I do agree with Dr Kumar that the TRH test can be troublesome, because we have had some excessive responses. However, in the majority of our patients there were no excessive responses, although, as Mr Walsh has shown, at the end of the cycle there was a difference. So we performed our tests between the fourth and eighth day after ovulation, generally about the fifth or the sixth day. In this way we avoided the difficulty that Mr Walsh had at the end of the cycle and this may account for the difference between his results and ours.

**Walsh**

That is possible.

**Gorins**

I must say I find Dr Kumar's reference to the dopamine-inhibition test very interesting.

**Hughes**

For those of you who are just surgeons like me, it might be helpful to point out that the relationship between pituitary stimulation with dopamine or domperidone and serum levels is that of maximal versus routine findings, rather like the old gastric test-meal, where there was maximal stimulation of the stomach with histamine and gastrin. I think this is a very exciting field—stimulating the pituitary maximally, rather than just taking serum levels which vary so much.

**Walsh**

I am not an expert on the prolactin secretion-stimulation test, but from the results that have emerged from the use of the test it seems that there may be an abnormal potential in the pituitary for secreting prolactin in some patients with benign breast disease. And

I think that the possible explanation may be, as I've said, an underlying abnormality of the oestrogens.

**Gorins**

Mr Walsh, did you examine the progesterone/oestradiol ratios and if so, what did you find?

**Walsh**

I looked at the figures in a preliminary way but I did not take them further than that. This is because the ratio of progesterone to oestradiol varies enormously, depending upon which part of the luteal phase one considers. The progesterone concentration can increase by a factor of 15 or 20, compared with its concentration in the follicular phase, and then it falls again. The oestradiol concentration may have a follicular phase level of 50 pg/ml and may go up to a luteal phase plateau of 150 pg/ml. So the ratio of the two will vary enormously in the individual, depending on where she is in the cycle. I was unable to find that the data produced anything worthwhile.

**Gorins**

I believe it is possible to smooth out the differences by taking the ratios at three points in the luteal phase, on the third, sixth and 10th days after ovulation.

**Walsh**

I find it difficult to establish the day of ovulation from basal body temperature recordings, on which I find it difficult, anyway, to place a great deal of trust. Even expert gynaecologists are known to have difficulty in estimating the day of ovulation from such recordings. This is why we didn't use this method to calibrate our data; instead, we calibrated the data by reference to the day of menstruation.

**Kumar**

The luteal phase we are talking about is a very artificial luteal phase if we take it just from basal body temperature or from the time of menstruation. Ovulation doesn't occur just 14 days before menstruation; it varies from the fifth to the 20th day. For this reason one needs to be sceptical about a defined luteal phase.

**Gorins**

Mr Kumar makes a good point. However, although quite often the luteal phase is of short duration, sometimes less than 10 days, in the majority of our cases, the luteal phase was of normal duration, between 10 and 14 days. Ovulation was measured by the elevation in temperature, and we find this easy and not very expensive to do. For us this is an important test.

**Kumar**

In most gynaecology departments, it is the LH surge which is used.

**Gorins**

We find the temperature test easier. The LH surge is difficult because it is very short and you have to do many tests to find it.

**Hughes**

These points certainly emphasize the importance of protocols in carrying out studies.

**Mansel**

I want to be slightly provocative. The two sets of data presented are completely different. If one looks at the Mauvais-Jarvis data, the standard errors do not even reach the normal range. One assumes the classification in France is fairly equivalent, so how are the completely different findings explained? Would Professor Gorins like to comment?

**Gorins**

I do not have the explanation. I want to say that some of us find an imbalance and some of us do not. Some find a luteal inefficiency, like Mauvais-Jarvis, and some do not find a progesterone disorder, like Mr Walsh and myself. For oestradiol, the position is the same. Although I have no explanation, I think the trouble is that benign breast disease does not arise from a basic hormonal disorder.

# Value of fine-needle aspiration cytology in the diagnosis of benign breast disease

HELEN L. D. DUGUID

*Cytology Unit, Department of Pathology,*
*Royal Infirmary, Dundee, Scotland*

Cytological diagnosis of malignancy by fine-needle aspiration biopsy was developed in Sweden where it has been practised since the early 1950s. It is quick, cheap, usually painless and can be carried out as an out-patient procedure. In the 1970s many articles appeared in the world literature discussing its value in the diagnosis of breast cancer and, although opinions at first varied from the sceptical to the enthusiastic, it is now generally accepted to be, in skilled hands, a useful and accurate method of diagnosis.

I propose to discuss the value of aspiration cytology in the diagnosis and management of the various types of benign breast disease, which in the Dundee Breast Clinic, amount to over 80 per cent of the cases requiring a pathological diagnosis.

Table 1 details the clinical diagnosis of 1083 women in whom fine-needle aspiration was carried out.

*Table 1*
*Dundee Breast Clinic: clinical diagnoses, January 1978–June 1980*

| Diagnosis | No. cases | |
|---|---|---|
| Benign breast disease | | |
|     Cyst | 234 | |
|     Dominant lump | 294 | |
|     Thickening | 373 | |
|     Total | 901 | (83%) |
| Carcinoma | | |
|     Operable | 131 | |
|     Inoperable | 51 | |
|     Total | 182 | (17%) |

*Benign Breast Disease, Edited by M. Baum, W. D. George, and L. E. Hughes, 1985: Royal Society of Medicine International Congress and Symposia series No. 76, published by The Royal Society of Medicine.*

In the Dundee Breast Clinic we carry out fine-needle aspirations on all palpable breast masses and give immediate provisional findings, using a rapid staining method which is mainly used in haematology and gives staining results similar to the Romanowsky stains (Duguid *et al.* 1979). At least two smears are made from each aspiration and the final report is made later, after examination of the second smear by the more sensitive Papanicolaou method.

Table 2 compares the cytological findings with the final clinical diagnosis.

*Table 2*

*Dundee Breast Clinic: cytological findings and final clinical diagnoses,*
*January 1978–June 1980*

| Cytological findings (Papanicolaou grading) | Total cases | Final clinical diagnosis | |
|---|---|---|---|
| | | Benign breast disease | Carcinoma |
| Unsatisfactory (class 0) | 124 | 112 (12%) | 12  (7%) |
| Normal/hyperplastic (class 1–2) | 777 | 764 (85%) | 13  (7%) |
| Suspicious (class 3) | 36 | 22  (2·4%) | 14  (8%) |
| Highly suggestive/positive (class 4–5) | 146 | 3  (0·3%) | 143 (79%) |
| Totals | 1083 | 901 | 182 |

## Methods of reporting

(See Table 2.)

### Unsatisfactory (class 0)
In our cytology reports we always evaluate the number of epithelial cells and the amount of stroma present. If the purpose of the report is to indicate merely the presence or absence of malignancy, then all samples which do not contain epithelial cells are classified as unsatisfactory. This was our original method of reporting but, with experience, we have learned that some breast masses consist almost entirely of fibrous connective tissue. Therefore, if malignancy is not clinically suspected and the aspiration is good, that is, if much stromal tissue is obtained, with few or no epithelial cells, we now provide a descriptive report and give it a class 1 classification.

### Normal (class 1–2)
The value of a class 1–2 report depends very much on the skill of the surgeon. He must use the point of the needle as a probe and after reaching an area of increased density, apply negative pressure and gently rotate the needle and move the point backwards and forwards in order to loosen the tissue. If necessary, three different areas of the mass may be sampled before withdrawing the needle. Equally important is the preparation of thin, evenly spread smears, as thick 'lumpy' smears cannot be evaluated with confidence.

### Positive (class 4–5)
At the other end of the scale there is the positive report indicating the presence of cells

with large nuclei, showing some variation in size with large multiple or irregular nucleoli and either poor cohesion or irregular arrangement. The number of false positive reports decreases with increasing experience, but very occasionally in benign lesions there is such a degree of epithelial hyperplasia with atypical features that a positive diagnosis is given. In cases where the cytology is definitely positive and the carcinoma is inoperable, we do not consider that an open biopsy is justified. When a mastectomy is considered necessary, we still always perform a frozen-section biopsy in order to rule out the rare possibility of a false-positive report.

### Suspicious (class 3)

Reports in this very interesting category are made in about 2·4 per cent of benign lesions and about 8 per cent of malignant lesions.

A certain number of suspicious reports are unavoidable. In benign breast disease, fibroadenomas showing marked epithelial hyperplasia can usually be diagnosed with confidence by the identification of typical bipolar stromal cells, but sometimes a class 3 suspicious report must be given. Mastopathy with atypical epithelial hyperplasia can produce suspicious large epithelial cells, with multiple nucleoli and showing poor cohesion. Here, a suspicious report is important as it suggests the possibility of eventual carcinoma; biopsy is required and careful follow-up.

## Pathological diagnosis and findings

Tables 3 and 4 detail the pathological conditions which can give characteristic cytological findings and the age groups at which these conditions are most commonly found (Melcher *et al.* 1981).

Cytologically a diagnosis of fibroadenoma is suggested by a specimen which is highly cellular and in which normal or hyperplastic duct cells are seen in conjunction with oval naked nuclei, probably derived from the myoepithelium. When these occur in pairs, they are called sentinel cells and are practically diagnostic of fibroadenoma.

Table 3

*Dundee Breast Clinic: pathological diagnosis and age of maximum incidence, January 1978–June 1980*

| Pathological diagnosis | Age of maximum incidence | | | | |
|---|---|---|---|---|---|
| | 15–24 years | 25–34 years | 35 years, menopause | Peri-menopausal | Post-menopausal |
| Fibroadenoma | + + | + | | | |
| (Mainly fibrosis) | | + + | | | |
| Mastopathy | | | | | |
| (Mainly epithelial hyperplasia) | | | + + | | |
| (Mainly cyst formation) | | | | + + | |
| Duct papilloma | | | | | |
| (nipple discharge) | | | | | + |

Table 4
Dundee Breast Clinic: pathological findings and age of maximum incidence,
January 1978–June 1980

| Pathological findings | Age of maximum incidence (years) | | |
|---|---|---|---|
| | 35 | 35–50 | 50 |
| Fat necrosis | + | + | + + |
| Puerperal mastitis | + + | | |
| Duct ectasia/periductal mastitis | | + | + + |
| Palpable lymph node in axillary tail | + | + | + |

If in addition to duct cells, foam cells, apocrine cells and scanty oval naked nuclei are seen, a benign mastopathy is suggested, the exception being the largely fibrotic lesions in which masses of stroma only are aspirated.

Breast cysts produce degenerate cellular material with masses of foam cells or papillary aggregates of duct or apocrine cells.

We have found that fat necrosis and duct ectasia, clinically often thought to be suspicious of malignancy, are conditions in which aspiration cytology will give the correct diagnosis. In fat necrosis, degenerate fat cells, polymorphs, histiocytes and scanty giant cells are seen in a blue-staining background containing lacunae, presumably due to dissolved lipid (Melcher et al. 1981). In duct ectasia, lymphocytes, plasma cells and histiocytes are found along with scanty foam cells and foreign body giant cells. Hyperplastic duct cells and histiocytes may have 'active' nuclei with nucleoli and must be distinguished from tumour cells.

In breast abscess, duct cells may show degeneration or hyperplasia with leucocytes and histiocytes and the diagnosis of a palpable lymph node is cytologically easy.

## Summary

Fine-needle aspiration cytology gives a correct diagnosis in 85 per cent of cases of benign breast disease, but some aspirations are unsatisfactory, others give suspicious reports and very occasionally, a false positive report is given. The results are not so clear cut as those of open biopsy. What then is its value?

In the Dundee Breast Clinic, we assess separately the three methods of out-patient diagnosis—physical examination, breast aspiration and mammography. If the breast aspiration is reported as unsatisfactory, it is either disregarded or immediately repeated and the detection of unsatisfactory aspirations is one of the values of the rapid provisional report. If all three methods point to a benign diagnosis, the patient is reassured, but an appointment is always made for follow-up examination.

In inflammatory conditions or fat necrosis, cytology can give a correct diagnosis where clinically the findings are considered to be suspicious of malignancy, but with these exceptions, early hospital admission for frozen-section biopsy is arranged when any one of the three methods of diagnosis gives either a suspicious or positive result.

Used in this way, cytology is a safe method of diagnosis and is of considerable value in the management of benign breast disease. Comparison with the other methods of diagnosis during the last six years has resulted in increasing reliance on its accuracy and it greatly reduces the number of cases which otherwise would have to be admitted to hospital for open biopsy.

## References

Duguid, H. L. D., *et al.* (1979). *Brit. Med. J.,* **2**, 185–7.
Melcher, D. H., *et al.* (1981). In *Recent advances in histopathology* (eds P. P. Anthony and R. N. H. MacSween), No. 11, pp. 263–280. Churchill, London.

## Discussion

### O'Higgins

I would like to ask Dr Duguid to comment on the role of cytology in patients whose cysts are not bloodstained. We have done this in the past, but no longer do so. Secondly, would she please comment on the value of cytology in nipple discharges which are likewise non-bloodstained.

### Duguid

Well, we do still look at breast cysts because we're interested. Some breast cysts have no cells, some have a lot of papillary cells, and we want to know if there is a relationship with whether or not the cyst is going to recur. But if all you want to know is whether the cyst is benign or malignant, I do agree that examination of a non-bloodstained cyst is really a waste of time.

Likewise with the nipple discharges, we find cytology here not very helpful. If the discharge is bloodstained or serous, then we do think of a papilloma and we do examine the specimen very carefully; but I would say 90 per cent of the nipple discharges we get are either duct ectasia, where all you get is pasty material with no cells at all, or you get masses of phagocytic cells. So here again, unless the nipple discharge is serous or bloodstained, if you're just thinking in terms of benign or malignant, cytology isn't worth doing.

### Parbhoo

I use cytology extensively but I still find difficulty in getting adequate specimens from some patients with fibrocystic disease. Often the lesion is like crêpe rubber and I find that the needle may, in fact, be bending in it. Do you have any suggestions about improving the yield of the material we send?

Secondly, I would like to sound a note of caution. In the very small lesions that we subject to cytology, where there's a query about whether they are benign or malignant, one may destroy the lesion so that the subsequent paraffin section fails to show up a small carcinoma.

### Duguid

Well, this question of unsatisfactory smears is a difficult one. We find that unsatisfactory smears are obtained, as you say, from mainly fibrous tissue, and they can be very hard. Normally we use ordinary green-capped 21 gauge intravenous needles, but we do have a supply of larger, thicker needles, which are baby lumbar puncture needles; these are much better needles but they are rather expensive. These are the needles we use for the very hard lesions. Where we can get false negatives is with very big tumours, because if you use just an ordinary small needle you may aspirate only the area of surrounding oedema. So one thing to do, when you think the lesion is very hard or very rubbery, is to use a thicker needle made of better steel. Another thing to do, as a routine, is to wet the inside of the needle with a little heparin–saline solution, and this does prevent the cells from sticking to the inner surface of the needle. Also, it is important to blow the material on to the slide, and sometimes you don't get material until the fifth blow.

I haven't had any experience so far of destroying the lesion by fine-needle aspiration.

**Hughes**

Can we ask Mr Parbhoo how he diagnoses it once it's been destroyed? Have I missed something?

**Duguid**

We did have one case where a GP did an aspirate and when we repeated it we got nothing but foreign body giant cells.

**Parbhoo**

In a small number of patients I have diagnosed 3 mm carcinomas on aspiration cytology, but in some other cases where we've done aspiration cytology we've had difficulty in finding the carcinoma on frozen section. And only after about 20 sections of the area does one eventually find the carcinoma. I sounded the note of caution, because in these circumstances you may miss the tumour on frozen section in the theatre.

**Duguid**

I would say to this that it is a different thing feeling a lump when the patient is sitting up and can point to where the lump is, from when the patient is lying flat and anaesthetized, when it is sometimes remarkably difficult to find a tiny lump. Mr Preece, do you find that you sometimes have to inject a marker substance?

**Preece**

In respect of these very, very small lesions, one would think that perhaps one shouldn't contemplate frozen sections. One should have urgent paraffin histology, as has been advocated by almost all centres for the subclinical lesions. I don't know what you would feel about that Mr Parbhoo?

**Parbhoo**

I'm just referring to the palpable lesion that the patient would point to as a small pea-sized nodule. And what I'm saying is that it is probably better to take the whole lump out rather than do cytology on such a very small lesion.

# Session 2:

## CHAIRMAN'S SUMMARY

### L. E. HUGHES

*University Department of Surgery,*
*Welsh National School of Medicine, Cardiff, Wales*

I think Professor Baum pointed out very clearly the problems that arise from benign breast disease and we must not neglect them as we have in the past. We must look at all our own ideas right from the question of public education through to booking our theatres.

Mr Mansel emphasized how vital it is to use an accurate clinical assessment, not only in treatment but also if we're going to look at the aetiology of this condition.

Professor Gorins reminded us of the importance of thermography, something which we have perhaps turned aside too much; and if we do use it we must remember to use it in association with all the other data. As far as the hormonal background to this condition is concerned, I think we're looking through a glass darkly at the moment, but there are some glimmers of light. It seems as though there may be changes in oestrogen and prolactin right at the end of the cycle and that the pituitary control may be abnormal. And of course, the target organ hasn't been looked at very much. We've obviously got to do a lot more work on this because hormonal manipulation is so important from the therapeutic point of view. The aetiology has to be chased until we really have the answers. There must be a very careful assessment of protocol if we're going to make any further advance in this field.

Finally, Dr Duguid has shown us how important cytology is, how important it is that we take the specimen properly and how important it is that we make a proper smear. If we do all these things, we are able to see positive evidence of benign breast disease as well as negative evidence—that cancer is not present. I was particularly interested to hear about her work on periductal mastitis, because that certainly can be very easily diagnosed on cytology when it simulates cancer from a clinical point of view.

So again we have had a very useful session. I'd like to thank the audience for their questions and participation and our speakers for their excellent presentations.

*Benign Breast Disease, Edited by M. Baum, W. D. George, and L. E. Hughes, 1985: Royal Society of Medicine International Congress and Symposia series No. 76, published by The Royal Society of Medicine.*

# Session 3:
# Danazol—pharmacology in relation to benign breast disease

## CHAIRMAN'S INTRODUCTION

### M. BAUM

*King's College Hospital Medical School,
London, England*

We have learned this morning that we are not at all sure what benign breast disease is and then we learned that we are not sure what causes this disease. However, this afternoon we are going to learn how to treat it!

Without doubt one of the very few agents available which is promising and which we do use in the clinic is danazol. It is therefore appropriate that in the next two sessions we consider the pharmacology of danazol and then the very serious and critical evaluation of this therapeutic agent.

We will begin by inviting Dr Gordon Potts to give the first paper—a fitting introduction to the session because it was Dr Potts who led the team that, in 1959, discovered this very interesting pharmacological agent.

*Benign Breast Disease, Edited by M. Baum, W. D. George, and L. E. Hughes, 1985: Royal Society of Medicine International Congress and Symposia series No. 76, published by The Royal Society of Medicine.*

# Pharmacology of danazol

**G. O. POTTS**

*Sterling-Winthrop Research Institute,*
*Rensselaer, New York, USA*

The objective of this presentation is threefold: first, I shall present a brief overview of the hormonal profile of this novel steroid; second, I shall review the binding affinity of danazol at the level of the oestrogen, progestogen and androgen receptors; and lastly, I shall speak of the relationship of the central inhibitory activity of danazol at the level of the hypothalmic–pituitary axis in terms of LH and FSH output, as well as its hormonal receptor affinity, as this may relate to the treatment of fibrocystic breast disease.

Danazol (Fig. 1) was synthesized at the Sterling-Winthrop Research Institute. It is a member of a large series of heterocyclic steroids distinguished by the addition of the isoxazole moiety to the A ring of a steroid, in this case ethisterone.

Extensive studies in a variety of preclinical and clinical situations have established that danazol is an orally active pituitary gonadotrophin inhibitory agent, without effect on any of the other pituitary trophic agents. It has weak impeded androgenic activity, well characterized in laboratory animals; it has weak anabolic activity, manifested clinically in the modest weight gain seen in some sensitive patients; it is devoid of oestrogenic and progestational activity; and it has no glucocorticoid or mineralocorticoid activities.

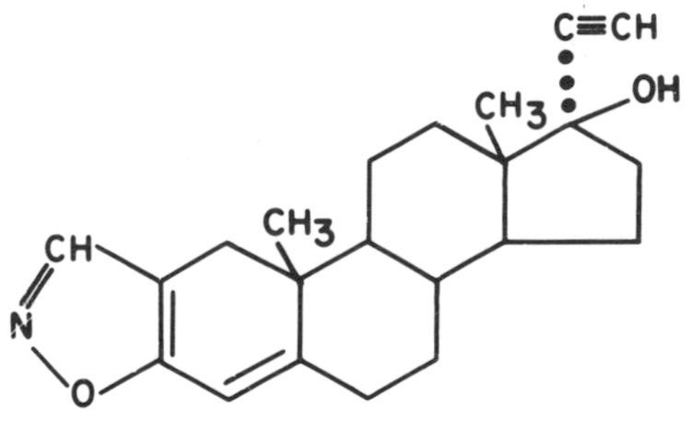

17α-Pregn−4−en−20−yno[2,3−d]isoxazol−17−ol

Fig. 1. *Molecular structure of danazol, a 2,3-isoxozol derivative of 17-ethinyltestosterone.*

*Benign Breast Disease, Edited by M. Baum, W. D. George, and L. E. Hughes, 1985: Royal Society of Medicine International Congress and Symposia series No. 76, published by The Royal Society of Medicine.*

In castrated immature female rats danazol, along with oestradiol, testosterone and dihydrotestosterone, suppresses the post-castration rise of both FSH and LH. Progesterone does not prevent the rise of either in this model (Eldridge *et al.* 1974).

Shane *et al.* (1978) demonstrated that danazol produced a dose-related decrease in LH in castrated female rats. After challenge with LHRH releasing factor it was established that danazol did not affect the release of LHRH (Fig. 2). There are two interpretations of these results: Shane *et al.* conclude that in all likelihood danazol has its effect at the level of the hypothalamus rather than the pituitary; I, on the other hand, favour the view that danazol acts directly on the pituitary to lower LH output. We have unreported data which provide convincing evidence that the administration of danazol to the intact female rat produces a suppressive effect on the pituitary–gonadal axis, associated with a significant increase in the pituitary content of gonadotrophins as indicated by bioassay.

Pedroza *et al.* (1978) presented evidence to the effect that the administration of danazol to immature male rats significantly blocked the response of the pituitary to LHRH (Fig. 3).

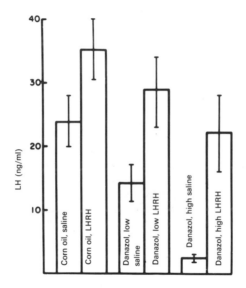

Fig. 2. *LH response by castrated female rats in indicated treatment groups.*

Franchimont and Cramilion (1977) demonstrated the reduction in the levels of FSH and LH in men and postmenopausal women after 15 days' treatment with danazol (Table 1). The release of FSH and LH in response to 25 µg of GnRH intravenously was significantly reduced by danazol in both normal men and women.

On the other hand, Asch *et al.* (1979) failed to show a blocking of the releasing factor in rhesus monkeys treated with 400 mg of danazol for seven days and then challenged with synthetic LHRH (Table 2).

In their early studies, Greenblatt *et al.* (1971) demonstrated the unequivocal suppression of the FSH–LH peaks in normally ovulating women following the administration of 800 mg daily. It is also worth noting that there was no suppression of the basal levels. Subsequently, Colle and Greenblatt (1976) presented evidence that while 100 mg danazol per day prevented the LH surge, 50 mg per day did not.

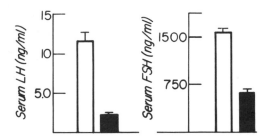

Fig. 3. Effect of treatment with danazol for 3 days on the pituitary-responsiveness to LHRH in immature male rats. Solid bars, danazol-treated; open bars, controls.

Table 1

Effect of danazol (600 mg per day for 15 days) on basal FSH and LH levels and on FSH and LH cumulative responses to an intravenous 25 μg GnRH injection

| Subjects and hormones | Basal levels (mIU/ml) | | | | Cumulative response to GnRH (mIU/2 h) | | | |
|---|---|---|---|---|---|---|---|---|
| | Before danazol | | After danazol | | Before danazol | | After danazol | |
| | Mean | S.E.M. | Mean | S.E.M. | Mean | S.E.M. | Mean | S.E.M. |
| Men (n = 5) | | | | | | | | |
| FSH | 4·62 | 0·73 | 2·42 | 0·53* | 413·2 | 63·3 | 262·5 | 63·2* |
| LH | 7·38 | 0·6 | 3·54 | 0·52† | 925·7 | 246 | 529 8 | 66·7* |
| Postmenopausal women (n = 5) | | | | | | | | |
| FSH | 49·6 | 8·21 | 24·2 | 7·7* | 2976 | 533 | 1310 | 331* |
| LH | 15·56 | 2·8 | 9·98 | 2·8† | 3279 | 624 | 1413 | 272* |

\* P < 0 05.
† P < 0·01.

Table 2

Effect of synthetic LHRH administration on LH plasma levels in three ovariectomized rhesus monkeys after treatment for 7 days with 400 mg danazol daily

| Time (min) | Control animals (ng/ml) | | | LHRF-treated animals (ng/ml) | | |
|---|---|---|---|---|---|---|
| | No. 1 | No. 2 | No. 3 | No. 1 | No. 2 | No. 3 |
| 0 | 1650 | 1060 | 2610 | 2430 | 1920 | 3820 |
| 30 | 1970 | 1780 | 2620 | 5300 | 3220 | 6990 |
| 60 | 2660 | 1740 | 3140 | 3800 | 3170 | 7090 |
| 80 | 2310 | 1380 | 2430 | 4040 | 2980 | 7400 |
| 120 | 3850 | 1250 | 1740 | 3750 | 3250 | 6910 |

Lauerson and Wilson (1976) demonstrated the inhibitory effect of danazol 200 mg daily on FSH and LH surges and on the menses, which did not occur until the drug was stopped.

In our own laboratory, Creange *et al.* (1979) investigating the mechanism of action of danazol, showed that it displaced labelled oestradiol from the pituitary, hypothalamus and hypothalamus minus the cortex (Table 3). The presumptive conclusion is

Table 3

Effect of danazol on distribution of [³H]oestradiol between plasma and cortex, pituitary and hypothalamus of ovariectomized rats

| | Tissue-specific activity/plasma-specific activity | |
|---|---|---|
| | Control | Danazol |
| Cortex | 0·22 ± 0·03 (16) | 0·36 ± 0·11  (15) |
| Pituitary | 6·12 ± 0·38 (16) | 3·22 ± 0·28* (15) |
| Hypothalamus | 0·80 ± 0·06 (15) | 0·53 ± 0·04* (14) |
| Hypothalamus (−) | 0·59 ± 0·06 (15) | 0·17 ± 0·02* (14) |

*Differs from mean of control group; $P < 0.001$.

reached that even though danazol is not oestrogenic, it binds to oestrogen receptors at the pituitary level, thereby modulating LH and FSH output.

In one of our early experiments (Table 4) we had demonstrated that danazol had an anti-oestrogenic effect in the castrated female rat. With danazol, cornified vaginal smears were reduced from 60 to 19 per cent, providing presumptive evidence of anti-oestrogenic activity.

Cook and Gibbs (1980) provided *in vitro* evidence that the marked binding competition between labelled oestradiol and unlabelled steroids established that compared with oestradiol, oestrone and oestrone-3-methyl ether, danazol is somewhat intermediate, with a weak inhibitory activity at about the level of that of oestriol. These authors demonstrated the same effects also in an ovine uterine cytosol *in vitro* experiment. Using the classical Clauberg assay, we have established the marked and dose-related anti-progestational activity of danazol (Table 5), and Barbieri *et al.* (1979) subsequently demonstrated the ability to danazol to displace tritiated progesterone from the progesterone receptor in rat uterine cytosol preparations (Fig. 4). This is an activity which is of ancillary value in the treatment of both endometriosis and benign breast disease.

In early studies, we investigated the anti-androgenic activity of danazol in the androgen-stimulated, castrated immature rat and showed that danazol will block the response to testosterone, particularly at lower levels (Table 6). Barbieri *et al.* (1979) established that danazol displaced tritiated dihydrotestosterone from the androgen receptor in a rat prostate cytosol preparation (Fig. 5), an *in vitro* confirmation of the anti-androgenic activity demonstrated *in vivo*.

Table 4

Effect of danazol with and without oestradiol in ovariectomized rats

| Treatment | Dose (mg (kg body weight)⁻¹d⁻¹) × 14 | No. rats | Body weight (g) Initial | Body weight (g) Final | Uterine weight (mg) | Vaginal cornification (percentage of total) |
|---|---|---|---|---|---|---|
| Control | — | 10 | 223 | 279 | 47·9 ± 1·6 | 0 |
| Danazol | 100 | 10 | 223 | 267 | 178·4 ± 7·2* | 9 |
| Danazol Oestradiol | 100 0·002 | 10 | 223 | 257 | 208·2 ± 7·6* | 19 |
| Oestradiol | 0·002 | 10 | 223 | 246 | 187·5 ± 5·7* | 60 |

*Significantly different from mean of control; $P < 0.001$.

Table 5

*Antiprogestational activity of danazol*

| Treatment | | No. rabbits | Endometrial response (mean ± s.e.) |
|---|---|---|---|
| Danazol (mg (kg body weight)$^{-1}$ d$^{-1}$) × 5 i.g. | Progesterone (mg (kg body weight)$^{-1}$ d$^{-1}$) × 5 i.m. | | |
| 0·0 | 0·0 | 5 | 0 |
| 0·0 | 0·2 | 5 | 4·0±0 |
| 12·5 | 0·2 | 5 | 3·6±0·2 |
| 25·0 | 0·2 | 5 | 3·2±0·5 |
| 50·0 | 0·2 | 5 | 0·6±0·4 |

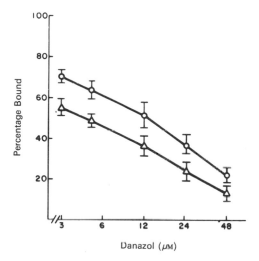

Fig. 4. *Semilogarithmic plot of danazol displacement of [³H]progesterone from the progesterone receptor of rat uterine cytosol.* △———△, *2nM progesterone;* ○———○, *10 nM progesterone. Apparent inhibition constant (K$_i$) for danazol is 6–9 µM (means±standard deviation; n=4).*

Punnonen and Lukola (1982) have shown that danazol competes with oestradiol, progesterone and dihydrotestosterone for receptors in a human uterine cytosol preparation, progesterone and dihydrotestosterone being more dramatically affected than the oestradiol (Fig. 6).

Nilsson *et al.* (1982) demonstrated the intermediate effect danazol has on the displacement of testosterone from sex hormone-binding globulin (SHBG) (Fig. 7).

Review of the literature on the preclinical and clinical pharmacology of danazol, i.e. of the hundreds of papers that have appeared during the last 20 years, leads us to the conclusion that the primary effect of danazol is mediated at the level of the hypothalamic–pituitary axis, suppressing the FSH–LH surge. This effect probably occurs because danazol is seen by the pituitary as an oestrogen and so binds to the oestrogen receptor. Thus we have the central activity of danazol, associated, as is well known, with a weak, impeded, androgenic activity.

*Table 6*

*Anti-androgenic activity of danazol in the castrated immature rat (seven rats per group)*

| Testosterone propionate (mg (kg body weight)$^{-1}$d$^{-1}$) × 10 s.c. | Ventral prostate (mg) ± S.E. | | |
|---|---|---|---|
| | Danazol (mg (kg body weight)$^{-1}$d$^{-1}$) × 10 i.g. | | |
| | 0·0 | 100 | 800 |
| 0·0 | 9·0 ± 1·4 | 17·3 ± 1·9 | 36·0 ± 2·1 |
| 0·7 | 67·4 ± 4·4 | 57·8 ± 7·5 | 56·1 ± 4·6 |
| 7·0 | 150·1 ± 9·0 | 128·5 ± 5·9 | 102·7 ± 8·2* |

\* Significantly different from the mean of the group treated with 7·0 mg of testosterone propionate alone; $P < 0·01$.

Other results which have appeared in the literature establish that danazol has, as a secondary and supporting mechanism of action, a marked capacity to compete with progesterone and testosterone at receptor sites.

There are thus two mechanisms—a central action and competition at receptor sites—precisely the mode of action one would wish to have in the treatment of endometriosis and fibrocystic breast disease.

So with danazol we have the capacity to alter the normal pituitary–gonadal–oestrogen–progesterone environment during the entire cycle. Although, as the Chairman correctly pointed out earlier today, we do not know precisely what the hormonal milieu is that produces benign breast disease, it is reasonable to assume that if one were to suppress the pituitary–gonadal axis and the oestrogen/progesterone levels, and in addition have the capacity to compete with oestrogen, progesterone and androgen at the receptor sites, one could anticipate the results that have in fact been seen in the clinic—reduction in pain, tenderness and nodularity. In the studies that we

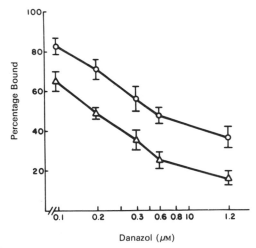

Fig. 5. *Semilogarithmic plot of danazol displacement of [$^3$H]dihydrotestosterone from the 8s androgen receptor of rat prostate cytosol.* △———△, *2 nM dihydrotestosterone;* ○———○, *7 nM dihydrotestosterone. Apparent inhibition constant (K$_i$) for danazol is 0·09 μM (means ± standard deviation; n = 4).*

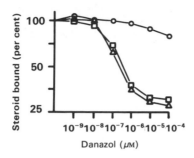

Fig. 6. *Competition of danazol for oestradiol* (○———○), *progesterone* (□———□) *and dihydrotestosterone* (△———△) *binding to the cytosolic uterine oestrogen, androgen and progesterone receptors. The cytosol used for progesterone receptor assay was pre-incubated for 1 h at 0 °C with a 100-fold excess of cortisol. All the values have been corrected for non-specific binding.*

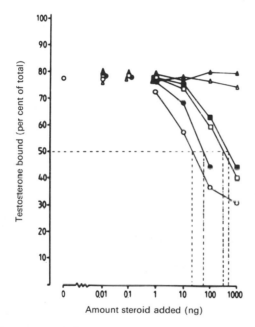

Fig. 7. *Displacement of [³H]testosterone from SHBG by different synthetic steroids. The amount of steroid necessary to reduce bound testosterone to 50 per cent of the total is indicated by dashed rules.* ○———○, *testosterone;* ●———●, *d-norgestrel;* □———□, *norethisterone;* ■———■, *danazol;* △———△, *medroxyprogesterone acetate;* ▲———▲, *tamoxifen.*

designed—in particular, the multicentre studies—and reported to the Food and Drug Administration in the United States, pain and tenderness tended to disappear in about six weeks. Nodularity tended to be more resistant and three to six months of danazol treatment was the time-frame for improvement.

Humphrey, in the USA, and some of the authors speaking this morning have postulated that in certain sub-sets, fibrocystic breast disease may be a continuum where yet to be well-characterized histopathological changes lead to a markedly increased risk of cancer. It may be that in due course, if appropriate studies are conducted over an adequate period of time, one might see a role for danazol in reducing the number of fibrocystic breast disease patients who go on to develop carcinoma.

## References

Asch, R., *et al*. (1979). *Obstet. Gynecol.*, **53**, 415.
Barbieri, R. L., *et al*. (1979). *Fertil. Steril.*, **31**, 182.
Colle, M. L., and Greenblatt, R. B. (1976). *J. Reprod. Med.*, **17**, 98.
Cook, D. B., and Gibb, I. (1980). *J. Steroid. Biochem.*, **13**, 1325.
Creange, J. E., *et al*. (1979). *Biol. Reprod.*, **21**, 27–32.
Eldridge, J. C., *et al*. (1974). *Biol. Reprod.*, **10**, 438–46.
Franchimont, P., and Cramilion, Cl. (1977). *Fertil. Steril.*, **28**, 814.
Greenblatt, R. B., *et al*. (1971). *Fertil. Steril.*, **22**, 102.
Lauerson, M. H., and Wilson, K. H. (1976). *Obstet. Gynec.*, **48**, 93–98
Nilsson, B., *et al*. (1982). *Fertil. Steril.*, **38**, 48.
Pedroza, E., *et al*. (1978). *Contraception*, **17**, 61.
Punnonen, R., and Lukola, A. (1982). *Horm. Metabol. Res.*, **14**, 167.
Shane, J. M., *et al*. (1978). *Fertil. Steril.*, **28**, 637.

## Discussion

### Baum

I'm not clear about the metabolism of danazol. Could I ask you, Dr Potts, about the way danazol is metabolized and whether any of its metabolites are active?

### Potts

We have looked at the metabolism of danazol thoroughly over the last 20 years and have detected no metabolite which would account in any way for the hormonal activity that we see. In other words, the metabolites are either inert or in such small quantities that they couldn't possibly be having the pharmacological effects. One of the things about this steroid which in my estimation is unique is that the isoxazole moiety stays intact in the metabolite situation, whereas the metabolism occurs in the rest of the molecule. So the metabolites, of which there are some 20, are all very minor. We have synthesized all the metabolites we have identified and they are either devoid of any activity or extremely weak.

### Gorins

I'd like to know what dosage of danazol is required to inhibit ovulation—100 mg, 200 mg or 400 mg per day? Often patients ask us if the compound is contraceptive.

### Potts

We have no reason to conclude from all of our clinical experience that we can produce anovulatory cycles 100 per cent of the time at doses less than 400 mg per day. We make no claim for contraceptive activity, and that is why in the prescribing information for danazol we suggest barrier contraceptive methods. In the early stages of danazol, we did run a contraceptive study and we found that at the level of 100 or 200 mg a day you are not going to see uniform anovulatory cycles. This leads me to mention that there is evidence that in mild cases of fibrocystic breast disease low dosages of danazol have produced rather striking relief of pain, tenderness and nodularity, which prompts one to conclude that if we are not blocking ovulation, we are not blocking the oestrogen/progestin aspect of the ovary, and so the antihormonal activity of danazol is coming into play at the level of the breast.

**Mansel**

You are probably aware that Ricardo Asch and Chamlis actually looked at what is probably a more relevant model, that was binding to MCF7 cancer cells, because that is probably as near to breast cells as we can get easily. They showed again what you have described, a differential response depending on the molarity of danazol. So it is obviously important for us to know what the concentration of danazol is in the patient's blood at a given dosage. Could you outline what sort of level one would find in a patient on 200 mg? $10^{-6}$? $10^{-9}$?

**Potts**

I don't have the figures with me, but that would be the general range. It is important to appreciate that with danazol, as with many other drugs, its concentration in the plasma may or may not be related to its binding affinity and half-life. Danazol *per se* has a long half-life in the plasma, but I am confident, from some of our unpublished data, that its affinity at the receptor level exceeds the plasma half-life, so, as good as the plasma level might be in indicating efficacy, one should not be surprised at having either receptor blockade or, indeed, central effect at points in time when blood levels are minimal or non-existent.

**Goebel**

Is there any change in prolactin receptors and size of the breast in cases of fibrocystic mastopathia?

**Potts**

In our multicentre study we reported a modest effect on breast size—a decrease.

**Parbhoo**

Following on the question put by Professor Baum, what is the major site of metabolism? Is it the liver? And secondly, if the levels of the metabolites are very low, does this mean that there is virtually no intrahepatic circulation? And thirdly, what is in fact the half-life?

**Potts**

The half-life is probably in the range 6–8 h in the plasma. The site of metabolism is the liver primarily. Which brings me back to the point I made earlier—once danazol binds at the level of the pituitary, it will exceed the plasma half-life, and that's where it has its activity.

# The effects of danazol on pulsatile LH release, basal LH and FSH serum levels, biphasic feedback of oestradiol and GnRH-induced gonadotropin release

## G. LEYENDECKER, L. WILDT AND P. BRAUN

*Department of Obstetrics and Gynaecology, University of Bonn, Bonn, West Germany*

Danazol, a synthetic derivative of 17α-ethinyltestosterone, has been used effectively for more than a decade for the treatment of endometriosis. Its mechanism of action, however, is still not well understood. Suppression of gonadotropin secretion, inhibition of ovarian steroidogenesis and interference with hormone action at the target tissues have all been proposed as possible modes of action of the drug. In this study, the effects of danazol on basal LH and FSH serum levels, pulsatile LH release, and response to oestradiol, progesterone and prolactin levels were examined in five healthy subjects during the follicular phase of the menstrual cycle. During a preceding control cycle the women had been subjected to the same procedures while taking no danazol.

During danazol administration, FSH serum levels were suppressed. This was, however, statistically significant only in blood samples taken at 20 min intervals for 6 h on days 3 and 4 of the cycle, and not in blood samples taken once daily. Basal LH levels and the number of LH pulses appeared to be reduced during danazol administration, while basal oestradiol and progesterone concentrations did not seem to be affected. Preliminary observations suggest, however, that LH and FSH levels and pulsatile LH release become significantly suppressed with time during long-term danazol administration. Basal prolactin levels did show a small but significant decrease when compared with control during danazol administration; the pituitary response to a single bolus injection of 100 µg GnRH on days 3, 4 and 8 of the cycle was the same as the controls. The inhibitory (negative feedback) effect of an increase of serum oestradiol produced by the injection of 5 mg EB on day 9 of the cycle was not altered by danazol treatment.

The stimulatory (positive feedback) action of oestradiol on gonadotropin secretion, however, was completely abolished in one subject and severely diminished in three subjects during danazol administration. In one subject, a normal increment in gonadotropin levels was observed after EB administration. Peak levels of gonadotropins were obtained earlier and the duration of the peak was shortened. This effect of

*Benign Breast Disease, Edited by M. Baum, W. D. George, and L. E. Hughes, 1985: Royal Society of Medicine International Congress and Symposia series No. 76, published by The Royal Society of Medicine.*

danazol on oestradiol-induced gonadotropin release is similar to that exerted by progesterone. In contrast, the increase in serum prolactin in response to EB administration was not altered by danazol treatment.

These data show that danazol administration reduces serum levels of FSH and LH, probably by reducing frequency of pulsatile gonadotropin secretion, interferes with the feedback effect of oestradiol on gonadotropin release in a similar way to progesterone, but does not interfere with the pituitary response to a single injection of GnRH. The effects of danazol on gonadotropin secretion may thus be sufficient to account for the anovulation produced by the drug. This does not exclude, however, the possibility that additional effects at the endometrial target cells are responsible for the effectiveness of this compound in the treatment of endometriosis.

## Discussion

**Baum**

If nothing else, that paper demonstrates the sophistication of modern endocrinology. We've come a long way in the last 10 years; we now recognize the importance of the diurnal variations in corticosteroid and prolactin levels; furthermore, instead of random blood samples, samples are taken in relation to the time of ovulation; and now we're really seeing chronobiology in action. I think the work is very exciting.

**Gorins**

The study is certainly a very interesting one and I like the way it demonstrated the disturbance of the feedback mechanism involving the hypothalamus and the hypophysis axis. Have you studied the problem of the peripheral effect also, that is to say, the effect on the ovaries? And did you try to give human menopausal gonadotropins to see if there was a response before danazol and during danazol? It seems to me that that is a question important to answer.

**Leyendecker**

I think that would be a very interesting study to carry out, but unfortunately we did not do it.

**Kumar**

I found your results very interesting indeed. My LH and FSH data after LHRH stimulation, in relation to cyclical mastodynia, have always puzzled me. The problem with my data, as I saw it, was the marked variation in LH and FSH secretion every day, every hour. It seems very worthwhile to consider such data in individual patients at hourly intervals in relation to the effect of danazol.

**Leyendecker**

We know from several studies, as far as negative feedback is concerned, that FSH is more sensitive to inhibition. This can be demonstrated during the normal menstrual cycle where, during the late proliferative phase, LH levels remain the same while FSH levels decline in the presence of rising oestradiol levels. So the differences in the effects of danazol on FSH and LH are very much consonant with physiological observations and studies on negative feedback in general.

**Baum**

Can I ask whether anyone has related the amplitude and frequency of these pulses of LH and FSH secretions, picked up on hourly observations, to benign breast disease?

**Leyendecker**

Perhaps one could see the effectiveness of the drug as far as suppression of the central system is concerned by studying after a while the pulsatility in the individual patient.

**Baum**

Well, in this session, two very clear messages have come across: first of all, Dr Potts has demonstrated clearly that danazol has a profound effect on some of the endocrinological pathways which, at least hypothetically, may be relevant to the nature of benign breast disease. And Professor Leyendecker has demonstrated how danazol might also be considered not just as a therapeutic weapon, but as a research tool for further helping us to dissect out the putative abnormalities in the endocrine control of breast development.

# Session 4:
# Danazol—clinical evaluations

## CHAIRMAN'S INTRODUCTION

### M. BAUM

*King's College Hospital Medical School,
London, England*

So far in this symposium we have considered why danazol should work in the management of benign breast disease. Now, as medicine is a scientific discipline having reasoned that it *should* work, we medical scientists must set out to determine whether it *does* indeed work. The next session is therefore of immediate clinical interest.

*Benign Breast Disease, Edited by M. Baum, W. D. George, and L. E. Hughes, 1985: Royal Society of Medicine International Congress and Symposia series No. 76, published by The Royal Society of Medicine.*

# A double blind trial of danazol in benign breast disease

R. E. MANSEL*

Department of Medicine, Division of Oncology,
The University of Texas, Houston, Texas, USA

## Introduction

I am going to describe to you today a controlled trial of danazol in painful benign breast disease which I carried out in conjunction with John Wisby, my research fellow at the time, at the Cardiff Mastalgia Clinic. We have heard here about the work of Ricardo Asch, an obstetrician and gynaecologist in America, who, with Robert Greenblatt, conducted all the preliminary studies on danazol (Asch and Greenblatt 1977). Although these two workers described good and very encouraging results in the resolution of lumps and pain in women with fibrocystic disease, all the studies were open and the results accumulated from the same set of patients, and we therefore felt that the final proof must come from a properly randomized controlled study. This is what we set out to do (Mansel *et al.*, 1982).

## Patients and methods

Twenty-eight patients were entered into the study, all with severe cyclical breast pain of at least six months' duration. (We chose to treat only the cyclical group because patients in this group had a greater severity of pain and because patients in the non-cyclical group had failed to respond to treatment with bromocriptine in a previous trial.) The trial was of the double blind, crossover type and each patient was randomized to start either on placebo or on danazol after a pre-trial observation month. The trial was six cycles long and the single crossover occurred at the mid-point. Most patients received 200 mg danazol daily, but the first six patients were given 400 mg daily to see the effect of the higher dose. These doses are lower than those usually recommended for the treatment of endometriosis. Assessment of response was made in each cycle in the late luteal phase, when symptoms were expected to be maximal, by the same clinician throughout the trial; additionally, patients carried out a self-assessment procedure.

The clinician assessed the response by interview and examination of the patient and recorded a score for breast tenderness and nodularity using a simple 1–3 scale (Fig. 1).

*Present appointment: Senior Lecturer, Hon. Consultant Surgeon, University Hospital of Wales, Cardiff, Wales.

*Benign Breast Disease, Edited by M. Baum, W. D. George, and L. E. Hughes, 1985: Royal Society of Medicine International Congress and Symposia series No. 76, published by The Royal Society of Medicine.*

## BREAST PAIN TRIAL CHART-CLINIC VISIT

HOSPITAL:                                    STUDY:

HOSPITAL REG. NO.:                           TRIAL NO.:

DATE:                                        NAME OR

                                             ADDRESSOGRAPH:

ASSESSMENT

1, 2, 3, etc.

*Clinical Assessment*

(a) TENDERNESS  ☐                (b) NODULARITY  ☐

   0 = Not examined                 0 = Not examined
   1 = No tenderness                1 = No nodularity
   2 = Some tenderness              2 = Some nodularity
   3 = Marked tenderness            3 = Marked nodularity

(c) RESPONSE TO TREATMENT  ☐      DESCRIPTIVE DIAGRAM

   0 = Not seen                      ▒ Diffuse granularity
   1 = Asymptomatic
   2 = Some improvement              ⁰₈⁰ Local nodules
   3 = No improvement
   4 = Worse

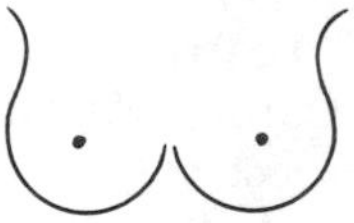

*Side effects*                    Table count: correct/incorrect

                                  Weight:

                                  BP:

Notes-e.g. blood taken, etc.:     Menstrual cycle: Regular/Irregular/None

*Fig. 1. Breast pain chart.*

    The patients completed a self-assessment form, marking their degree of pain (from 'none' to 'unbearable') on a visual linear analogue scale (Fig. 2); general symptoms were also covered in the same way. The forms were completed in a separate room, out of sight of the doctor, and filed away for analysis at the end of the trial. Scores of between 0 and 100 for each symptom were derived by measuring the length of the line from the left-hand point to the mark made by the patient. Since the figures produced were not discreet measurements, we used non-parametric statistics—the Wilcoxon signed ranks test—to analyse the results for significance.

    Of the 28 patients initially entered, six dropped out of the trial, three on danazol and three on placebo. We were interested to note that the drop-outs were divided equally between danazol and placebo, the implication being that the side effects of danazol were not as severe as we had been led to expect. One patient was excluded from analysis because the returned capsule count indicated that she was not taking the trial capsules as directed. Thus 21 patients satisfactorily completed all six cycles of the trial.

    The mean age of the patients was 30 years (typical of cyclical breast pain patients) and the patients weighed between 42 and 88 kg (Table 1). The mean duration of breast pain was more than four years, with a range of 1–13 years, again typical of the severe cases we treat.

Have you had any of the following symptoms or problems over the last 2 weeks?

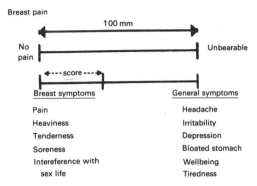

Fig. 2. Linear analogue form.

Table 1

Danazol trial—patient characteristics (n=28)

| | |
|---|---|
| Age | 30 ± 5 years (20–39) |
| Weight | 57 ± 10 kg (42–88) |
| Duration of symptoms | 4·1 ± 3·7 years (1–13) |

## Results

The results of the clinician's assessments are shown in Table 2. Since the maximum score was three, it will be seen that the pre-trial means for tenderness and nodularity were both high. Although there appeared to be a placebo response for tenderness (from 2·2 to 1·8), there was no response for nodularity. The scores for danazol for both tenderness and nodularity showed that the response was both marked and significant.

The results of treatment as assessed by the patient for breast tenderness, using the visual analogue scale, are shown in Fig. 3. The group randomized to start on placebo had a high pre-trial mean of more than 80. Placebo produced a fall to a mean of 60, but at the three-month crossover point a further clear improvement began on danazol and the improvement continued until the symptoms were virtually abolished. The effects of placebo treatment that were demonstrated clearly indicate that a double-blind trial is essential for a valid study to be produced. Patients who began with danazol had a large reduction in tenderness, from a pre-trial mean of 70 to a final level of 20. There was no further improvement when these patients crossed over to placebo and in fact there was some evidence of a return of symptoms after three months' placebo treatment.

There was thus agreement between clinician and patient that danazol significantly improves breast tenderness. A similar finding was reached for nodularity, but with a slower time-course.

Results were assessed also by counting the days of pain on each patient's pain chart (see the paper by Mansel in Session 2: 'Classification of mastalgia—the Cardiff

Table 2

Clinician's asessment—danazol trial (means±S.D.)

|  | Pre-trial | Placebo | Danazol |
|---|---|---|---|
| Tenderness | 2·22 ± 0·7 | 1·89 ± 0·7 | 1·18 ± 0·2* |
| Nodularity | 2·00 ± 0·5 | 2·04 ± 0·6 | 1·37 ± 0·4* |

*P < 0·05; paired 't' test.

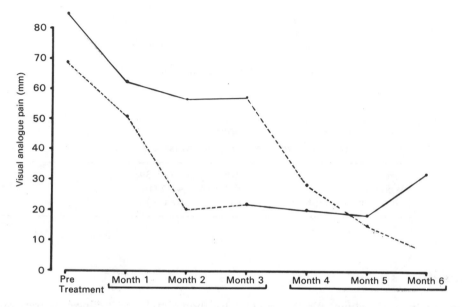

Fig. 3. Mean visual analogue score for tenderness. ●———●, placebo; ●－－－●, danazol.

system'). Danazol reduced an average of eight to 10 days of pain to about three days, regardless of treatment order (Fig. 4). Placebo had no effect and again there appeared to be some return of symptoms by the sixth month in the group which received danazol as the first treatment.

The most striking hormone results were those concerning progesterone (Table 3). Pre-trial levels were within normal limits and placebo had no significant effects. Danazol, on the other hand, lowered serum progesterone to follicular phase levels, regardless of the treatment order, suggesting that LH surges had been abolished and that the patients were not ovulating. In the placebo period, following the danazol treatment period, there was some recovery of the progesterone but not to pre-trial levels, indicating a carry-over effect of the drug.

As expected, disturbance of menstruation was the most common side effect, with 16 patients reporting some disturbance, six of whom had amenorrhoea. As many reports have suggested that the mild anabolic effect of danazol is a problem, we examined the side effect of weight gain. Although patients in the danazol group showed some weight gain, the increase was not significant (Table 4). This may well have been due to the lower dose that we used and to the fact that the trial protocol limited the patients

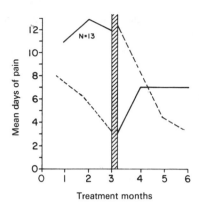

Fig. 4. Pain chart results. ———, placebo; ----, danazol; hatched area indicates crossover point.

Table 3

*Danazol trial—hormonal effects*

|  | Serum progesterone levels (ng/ml) | | |
|---|---|---|---|
|  | Pre-trial | Placebo | Danazol |
| Placebo first | 18·3 ± 17 | 26·3 ± 18 | 3·3 ± 2·1 |
|  | Pre-trial | Danazol | Placebo |
| Danazol first | 24·4 ± 17 | 1·8 + 1·2 | 10·1 ± 10·5 |

Table 4

*Danazol trial—side effects*

|  | Body weight (mean ± S.D.) (kg) |
|---|---|
| Pre-trial | 56·4 ± 11 |
| End of placebo | 56·0 ± 10 |
| End of danazol | 58·5 ± 11 |

'*t*' test, n.s.

to an upper weight maximum so preventing entry of obese women who seem to put on weight more easily on danazol.

## Conclusions

This study shows clearly that danazol significantly reduced breast tenderness and nodularity in a selected group of patients with severe cyclical mastalgia. Side effects occurred but at lower doses were relatively mild. Danazol is therefore a useful addition to our armamentarium for the treatment of severe benign breast disease.

## References

Asch, R. H., and Greenblatt, R. B. (1977). *Amer. J. Obstet. Gynecol.*, **127**, 130.
Mansel, R. E. *et al.* (1982). *Lancet* **i**.

# Xeromammographic changes associated with danazol therapy

## M. W. KISSIN*

*Northwick Park Hospital and Clinical Research Centre,
Harrow, Middlesex, England*

## Introduction

Despite widespread use of danazol in the management of breast pain, there is relatively little information concerning objective response to treatment. Most published trials have concentrated on subjective relief of symptoms (Mansel *et al.* 1982).

The aim of this study was to assess objective changes in xeromammography after danazol therapy, and to correlate structural change with symptomatic relief.

## Patients and methods

From January to August 1982, 16 women were studied. Each presented with cyclical breast pain of at least six months' duration, and of severity to interfere with their lifestyle. Five patients also had a history of recurrent breast cyst formation. No patient had received previous hormonal treatment for breast pain, or had been on an oral contraceptive pill in the preceding three years. The mean age was 43 years (range 23–60 years), and one patient was postmenopausal.

Danazol was given in the first instance for a period of 12 weeks, commencing at a daily dose of 600 mg. After four and eight weeks the daily dose was reduced to 400 mg and 200 mg respectively. Six patients were given 200 mg maintenance therapy for a further six to 12 weeks.

Xeromammography was carried out before commencement and after cessation of danazol. In an effort to limit radiation exposure, only two views were taken, both being in the negative mode. Care was taken to ensure that exposure and development conditions were identical in both sets of films. These were then read 'blind' by two independent observers, and differences in the degree of dysplasia graded either as no change, slight change or marked change.

Symptomatic response was assessed by questionnaire and interview, and clinical changes by examination of breast texture and size.

*\*Present appointment: Surgical Research Fellow, Royal Marsden Hospital, Fulham Road, London SW3, England.*

*Benign Breast Disease, Edited by M. Baum, W. D. George, and L. E. Hughes, 1985: Royal Society of Medicine International Congress and Symposia series No. 76, published by the Royal Society of Medicine.*

## Results

Complete symptomatic relief occurred in 12 patients (75 per cent), and partial relief was experienced by a further three. Only one patient reported no clinical improvement. The following side effects were noted: amenorrhoea, 60 per cent; weight gain (of less than 2 kg), 25 per cent; mood change, 18 per cent.

On examination a softening in breast texture was noted in 14 patients (88 per cent), a reduction in nodularity in eight patients (50 per cent) and a reduction in breast size in six patients (38 per cent).

Marked mammographic improvement was seen in four patients (25 per cent), and slight improvement in a further seven patients (43 per cent). All 11 patients with mammographic resolution experienced complete relief of breast pain and resolution of nodularity. Of those patients with no evidence of structural change, one had complete relief of symptoms, three had partial relief and one had no change.

### Case report 1

A 48-year-old mother of two presented with a five year history of severe cyclical breast pain. On examination there was marked nodularity. The pretreatment film (Fig. 1, left) shows moderate dysplasia particularly in the upper zone. After 12 weeks of treatment she experienced complete symptomatic relief and her breasts became softer and smaller. The post-treatment film (Fig. 1, right) shows slight mammographic resolution.

### Case report 2

A 42-year-old mother of one presented with a 12-month history of cyclical breast pain and a past history of recurrent breast cysts. On examination there was marked nodularity. The pretreatment film (Fig. 2, left) shows prominent sheets of dysplastic breast tissue. After 16 weeks of therapy she experienced complete symptomatic relief and the breasts were softer and smaller. The post-treatment film (Fig. 2, right) shows a marked softening and reduction in dysplasia, and a reduction in breast size. She had no further symptoms for 15 months.

## Comment

In this study structural improvement was seen in 68 per cent of patients after danazol therapy. Clinical improvement was reported in 94 per cent and in 75 per cent there was a good correlation between structural change and symptomatic response. These results are in close accordance with those reported by Asch and Greenblatt (1977) and Ouimet-Oliva et al. (1981). That structural changes are less marked than relief of symptoms may be attributed to danazol affecting the glandular more than the fibrous elements.

Mammographic resolution may be of significant value in the detection of small breast tumours previously obscured by sheets of dysplastic tissue. Danazol may, therefore, be useful in patients with high risk mammograms, particularly those with dysplasia persisting into the menopause.

## Acknowledgements

I would like to thank Mr A. E. Kark for permission to study his patients, and Dr J. D. Spencer for his assistance in interpretation of the xeromammograms.

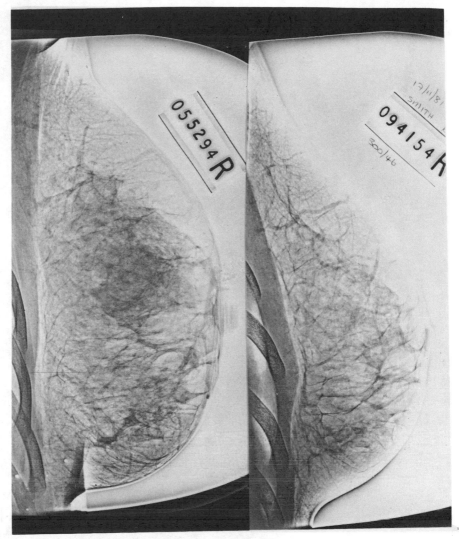

*Fig. 1. Case 1: pretreatment film (left) and post-treatment film (right).*

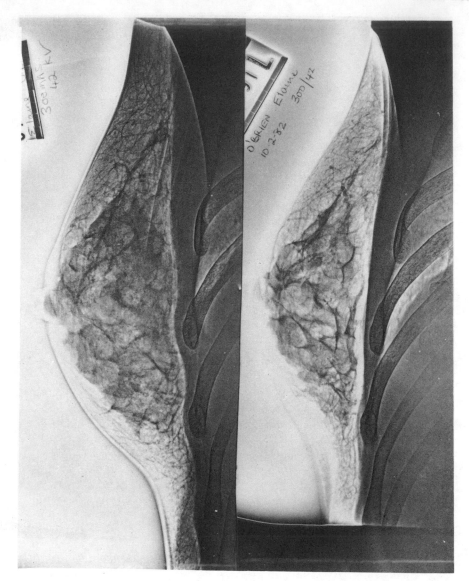

Fig. 2. Case 2: pretreatment film (left) and post-treatment film (right).

# References

Asch, R. H., and Greenblatt, R. B. (1977). *Amer. J. Obstet. Gynecol.,* **127**, 130–4.
Mansel, R. E., *et al.* (1982). *Lancet,* **i**, 928–31.
Ouimet-Oliva, D., *et al.* (1981). *J. Canad. Assoc. Radiol.,* **32**, 159–61.

# Comparison of danazol with tamoxifen, gestagen, acupuncture, local treatment and placebo: results in one thousand patients

## W. EGGERT-KRUSE, D. VON FOURNIER, U. LEGLER AND H. JUNKERMANN

*Department of Obstetrics and Gynaecology, University of Heidelberg, Heidelberg, West Germany*

Our studies of mastopathy and of its treatment have been carried out at the Heidelberg University Breast Clinic, part of the Department of Obstetrics and Gynaecology.

In our clinic we provide a full range of examination techniques, including mammography, electronic thermography, liquid crystal thermography, fine-needle cytology, drill biopsy and ultrasound scan. Surgical techniques conducted at the clinic include the cosmetic and plastic reconstruction of the breast, and postoperative radiotherapy and chemotherapy are offered.

About 33 per cent of our patients are referred for further investigation by private doctors from a large area around Heidelberg, but in non-selected samples, we have found mastopathy generally occurs in about 21 per cent but only about 6 per cent need treatment.

The mild forms of mastopathy seen include breast symptoms associated with premenstrual syndrome and oedematous swelling with pain. Slight objective X-ray changes may be seen and mild changes also on ultrasonography and thermography. Mastopathy is defined as severe when changes on mammography and/or on other examinations are found to be marked or severe and when the signs and symptoms are not related to the menstrual cycle.

The results of various treatments for mastopathy were examined and compared in prospective and retrospective studies during the years 1965–82.

Retrospectively, we examined the effects of local therapy (anti-inflammatory agents with 70 per cent alcohol) compared with oral gestagens and with auriculo-acupuncture, and the effects of the anti-oestrogen tamoxifen compared with danazol. Tamoxifen was administered at a dosage of 10 mg daily throughout the cycle, except for a five day pause during menstruation; danazol was given at three different dose levels—100 mg, 200 mg or 400 mg daily—and again medication was interrupted during a menstrual period.

**Figures 1, 2 and 3 in this paper are to be found in the colour section at the end of the symposia.**

*Benign Breast Disease, Edited by M. Baum, W. D. George, and L. E. Hughes, 1985: Royal Society of Medicine International Congress and Symposia series No. 76, published by the Royal Society of Medicine.*

Table 1

*Results of various treatments for mastopathy (subjective improvement; retrospective study, 1965–82)*

| Treatment regimen | *n* | Symptom-free (per cent) | Improved (per cent) | Total response (per cent) |
|---|---|---|---|---|
| Local therapy | 350 | 15 | 38 | 53 |
| Gestagens | 270 | 45 | 31 | 76 |
| Auriculo-acupuncture | 130 | 48* | 36* | 84* |
| Tamoxifen | 55 | 38 | 43' | 81 |
| Danazol | 153 | 43 | 34 | 77 |

*Therapy effect was time-limited.

Results of the analysis are shown in Table 1. Results achieved with local therapy, gestagens and auriculo-acupuncture varied from 53 to 84 per cent improvement in total subjective complaints; tamoxifen and danazol both achieved a total response rate of about 80 per cent. More patients receiving danazol at a dose of 200 mg daily became symptom-free than those on a dose of 100 mg daily.

In patients who did not respond to one or other of the first three forms of therapy, either tamoxifen or danazol was generally found to be nevertheless successful. In cases of severe mastopathy, an objective response of the mastopathic lesion was frequently found only with danazol and tamoxifen. Of all forms of therapy, danazol at a dosage of 200 mg daily was found to be the most effective.

In a three- to six-month prospective study, in which most patients (24 out of 35) received 200 mg danazol daily, danazol proved to be slightly more effective than tamoxifen (Table 2). Maximum effectiveness was achieved after three months of therapy; essentially, no further improvement was observed after an additional three

Table 2

*Prospective comparison of tamoxifen and danazol in three to six months of treatment for mastopathy (1981–2)*

| | Symptom-free (per cent) | Improved (per cent) | No response (per cent) |
|---|---|---|---|
| Tamoxifen (*n* = 35) | | | |
| Patients' reports | 42 | 46 | 12 |
| Clinical examination | 6 | 58 | 36 |
| Danazol (*n* = 35) | | | |
| Patients' reports | 67 | 27 | 6 |
| Clinical examination | 3 | 55 | 42 |

months of treatment. Of the two therapeutic regimens, danazol again was found to be the most effective. Sixty-seven per cent of the patients treated with danazol became symptom-free (tamoxifen 42 per cent) and a further 27 per cent were markedly improved (tamoxifen 46 per cent). Only 6 per cent of the danazol patients showed no response to treatment.

Side effects are listed in Table 3. Severe side effects (necessitating termination of therapy) were seen in 8 per cent of the danazol patients and 6 per cent of those receiving tamoxifen. Fifty-one per cent of the danazol patients had no side effects at all compared with 34 per cent of the tamoxifen patients. Of the marked side effects, weight gain, amenorrhoea and hair loss were seen in both groups of patients. Four danazol patients complained of hoarseness.

Danazol side effects occurred at daily dosages of both 100 mg and 200 mg; even at the lower dose level, acne, hoarseness and amenorrhoea were noted, whilst similar side effects were seen also at the higher dose level, with the addition of fatigue and hair loss. Of the three danazol patients with severe side effects who had to be withdrawn from therapy, one was receiving 100 mg and two 200 mg daily.

Mammograms of a patient with severe dense fibrocystic disease before and after danazol treatment are shown in Fig. 1. After six months' treatment with danazol 200 mg daily, reduction in the size and density of the breast was observed and improved radiographic transparency, confirming the improvement seen on clinical examination.

The effects of danazol are also seen in pre- and post-treatment thermograms shown in Fig. 2. These illustrate massive hyperthermia with an irregular vascular pattern, responding to six months of danazol 200 mg daily. Breast temperature is considerably reduced and the pathological vascular pattern has become normal.

Figure 3 shows the improvement demonstrated by mammography in a patient receiving 10 mg tamoxifen daily for a period of six months. A marked reduction in density is clearly seen.

*Table 3*

*Prospective comparison of side effects of tamoxifen and danazol in three to six months'*
*treatment for mastopathy (1981–2)*

| Severity of side effects | Tamoxifen ($n = 35$) | Danazol ($n = 35$) |
|---|---|---|
| None | 34 per cent | 51 per cent |
| Mild | 40 per cent: hot flushes 7; acne 3; nausea 3; spotting 1 | 25 per cent: acne 4; irregular menstruation 3; nausea 2 |
| Marked | 42 per cent: fatigue 4; weight gain > 4 kg 3; hot flushes 2; amenorrhoea 2; hair loss 1; pruritus vulvae 1; ovarian cysts 1; decrease of libido 1 | 48 per cent: weight gain > 4 kg 7; hoarseness 4; amenorrhoea 3; marked acne 1; hair loss 1; fatigue 1 |
| Severe (interruption of therapy necessary) | 6 per cent: nausea and gastric pain 2 | 8 per cent: nausea/depression 2; gastric pain 1 |

*Note:* Comparison of three and six months' therapy showed no increase in side effects. Some patients experienced multiple side effects.

## Conclusions

Following a retrospective review of patients treated for mastopathy, a prospective study has shown that a marked improvement in subjective symptoms of more than 80 per cent can be achieved with danazol and tamoxifen. The impressive therapeutic effects of these agents can be demonstrated by mammography, thermography and other investigating techniques.

The importance of these two drugs, in spite of the high incidence of side effects, is demonstrated by the fact that they are found to be effective in a high proportion of patients who have not responded to other forms of treatment.

# Experience with danazol in the UCH Breast Clinic: an open study

## N. B. SHAIKH

*University College Hospital,
London, England*

## Introduction

The two major problems that a clinician faces in breast disease are carcinoma of the breast and breast pain. Breast cancer is ultimately lethal in the majority of cases, and the state of our knowledge—its understanding and management with a view to cure—still unsatisfactory. The other problem which bothers the patient the most is breast pain. In recent years there has been greater awareness of problems associated with benign breast disease and it appears that the problem is now being given more serious attention. Non-cyclical pain is probably more amenable to treatment than cyclical pain. As elsewhere, we at UCH have tried many sorts of treatment, from reassurance to the use of vitamin E, diuretics, non-steroidal anti-inflammatory analgesics, ordinary analgesics and the prolactin inhibitor bromocriptine. As is well known, except for bromocriptine, none of the agents mentioned has given consistently acceptable results. Bromocriptine has fairly severe side effects but probably still has a place in the treatment of women with severe cyclical mastalgia. Following reports on the value of danazol in the management of mastalgia, we at UCH began to use the drug and have used it now for nearly two years, treating, on average, 60–70 patients with severe or moderately severe mastalgia each year.

## Magnitude of the problem

At UCH Breast Clinic 700–800 new cases are seen in the course of a year. An analysis of one year's new cases is shown in Fig. 1. In nearly 30 per cent the principal complaint was of pain, either unilaterally or in both breasts. Twelve per cent of the total had non-cyclical pain, and these include those with Tietze's syndrome, duct ectasia with periductal mastitis and sclerosing adenosis. Seventeen per cent had cyclical breast pain with varying degree of nodularity. Out of these, nearly half (8 per

**Figures 5, 6 and 7 in this paper are to be found in the colour section at the end of the symposia.**

*Benign Breast Disease, Edited by M. Baum, W. D. George, and L. E. Hughes, 1985: Royal Society of Medicine International Congress and Symposia series No. 76, published by the Royal Society of Medicine.*

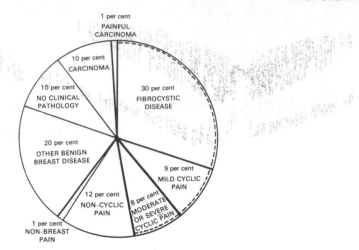

*Fig. 1. Analysis of 736 new cases seen at UCH Breast Clinic in one year.*

cent) had pain of severe or moderately severe degree, and it was patients from this group that were included in this open danazol study.

## Materials and methods

Fifty-seven cases of severe or moderately severe mastalgia were included in this study. All were premenopausal women, and seven had had a hysterectomy with preservation of ovaries. All were between the ages of 21 and 42 years. Each patient was started on danazol 100 mg twice daily. In two patients who responded well but who had troublesome side effects we reduced the dose to 100 mg once daily. All patients over the age of 30 years had mammography performed along with the other routine investigations before starting danazol. Every patient was examined at the end of each month and assessed for changes in their symptoms of pain and tenderness and the clinical signs of nodularity. Side effects were assessed at the same time. No patient was allowed any concurrent hormonal contraceptive. Each patient was asked if she had complete relief or significant improvement (indicating no interference in normal activity and no further need for analgesia), or no change (which included very little change or uncertainty on the part of the patient's own assessment).

Lumpiness or patches of coarse nodularity were assessed by comparing with previous markings on rubber stamp diagrams of breasts. For the sake of convenience, clinical coarse nodularity was classified in degrees. First degree was coarse nodularity, which is found in the majority of cases and is the commonest in supra-areolar regions and in the upper outer quadrant including the axillary tail. Diffuse lumpiness or nodularity in almost all the quadrants was labelled as third degree. Second degree was that falling in between, for example, a couple of patches in infra-areolar regions or other parts along with upper outer quadrant patchiness or supra-areolar lesions (Fig. 2).

## Results

Of the 57 patients, four stopped taking danazol because of severe side effects. Two of

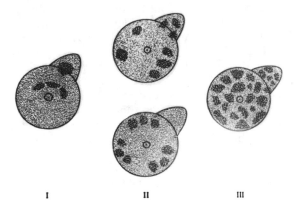

I                II                III

*Fig. 2.  Coarse nodularity classification.*

them developed severe nausea and vomiting and the other two developed migraine-like headaches. Neither of these patients had a previous history of migraine or headache. Fifty-three patients completed the minimum course of three months (Fig. 3). Twenty-one patients experienced complete relief of pain and 18 experienced a significant improvement in their symptoms. Fourteen patients either had no improvement at all, admitted to only marginal improvement or were uncertain of their own

RESPONSE OF SYMPTOMS TO DANAZOL

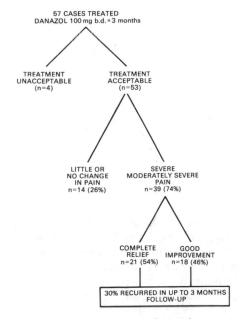

*Fig. 3.  Patient response to danazol treatment.*

assessment. Those with complete relief had remarkable resolution of nodularity as well. Patients with diffuse nodularity of third degree had come down to second or first degree of nodularity. Of those with first or second degree nodularity, almost half had complete resolution of the clinical signs of nodularity. The 18 patients who had a significant improvement also showed reduction in the nodularity of their breasts, but in the main the nodularity had become softer. In two of these patients, after the resolution of nodularity, fibroadenomas became apparent which were subsequently removed. In one 29 year old patient, after the disappearance of nodularity in the upper outer quadrant, a small, firm, discreet lump remained after the first month of treatment. This was thought to be suspicious and excision biopsy of the lump proved it to be carcinoma.

An interesting group of patients included in the study were those who had had a hysterectomy with preservation of ovaries. These patients were under the age of 42 years and had complained of severe or moderately severe pain with lumpiness of their breasts. Although they had no periods, on very close questioning one could elicit a cyclical pattern of pain. Five of the seven patients in this group responded with complete relief or significant improvement in their pain and marked reduction in the nodularity of their breasts.

It appears that the shorter the length of history of complaints, the more satisfactory is the response (Fig. 4). Of the seven patients with a three-month history of severe or moderately severe breast pain and nodularity, six responded. Of those with a six-month history, 11 out of 13 responded. Of those with a one-year history, only four out of seven responded. Also, the more severe the pain and symptoms, the better was the response; and the higher the dose, the better the response but the more severe the side effects as well.

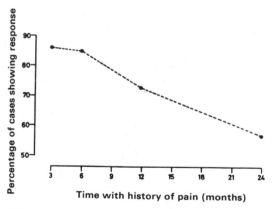

*Fig. 4. Effect of length of history of pain on treatment response.*

We have been able to follow up those cases who responded satisfactorily, so far for up to six months after stopping the drug. Two months after stopping the drug there was one recurrence; after three months there were five recurrences and after six months there were nine recurrences. Thus, six months following cessation of danazol treatment, 15 out of 39 patients (38 per cent) who had responded satisfactorily had returned with recurrence of their symptoms (Fig. 1), although in about half of them the symptoms were not as severe as they had been in the beginning. In one, the recurring symptoms were far more severe than originally. Those who had recurrence

Table 1

*Side effects of danazol treatment*

| Side effect | Patients |
|---|---|
| Weight gain > 2 kg | 17 (30 per cent) |
| Menstrual disturbance | 19 (33 per cent) |
| Nausea and vomiting | 4 (7 per cent) |
| Skin rash | 3 (5 per cent) |
| Headaches: severe | 2 (4 per cent) |
| Headaches: mild | 1 (2 per cent) |
| Lethargy and weakness | 4 (7 per cent) |

responded to danazol again when they were restarted on the drug. Two of the patients in the post-hysterectomy group had two recurrences of symptoms each and on both occasions their pain and nodularity responded to another course of danazol. In some cases where nodularity was shown on physical examination to have been reduced, mammography was repeated and confirmed lesser density and lesser nodularity of the breasts (Figs 5–7).

## Side effects

Side effects are listed in Table 1. Seventeen patients (30 per cent) gained weight of more than 2 kg. Disturbances of menses (amenorrhoea, scanty or irregular periods), which occurred in 19 patients (33 per cent), was complained of more by those who had not responded than those who had responded to the treatment. Troublesome nausea and vomiting was reported by four patients (7 per cent). A rash on the face and on the body was reported by three patients (5 per cent) but, as it was not troublesome in the case of two patients, they continued to take the drug. One of these, however, stopped at the end of the second month. Danazol appeared to precipitate migraine in two patients with no previous history of the condition. One patient reported a mild headache and four reported a feeling of weakness, lethargy, flushes and a feeling of not being well.

## Conclusion

Danazol is definitely a useful agent, effective in relieving mastalgia and nodularity in the majority of cases. The shorter the history, the more effective is the response. The side effects are acceptable and not unreasonably disturbing. The rate of recurrence of symptoms, however, appears to be high and it seems to be time-related, the longer the follow-up, the greater the recurrence rate. One group in which danazol may be particularly useful is that of post-hysterectomy mastalgia patients. Some discrete lumps may become clinically detectable after the resolution both of pain and nodularity, and this might reveal a carcinoma or fibroadenoma, or a particularly painful 'trigger spot', the excision of which may well bring relief to the patient.

For the future we need more information to allow us to select those patients likely to respond to danazol therapy, and the possible role of maintenance therapy in those who relapse after successful treatment requires some evaluation. Also, lower dosages of danazol and the stages of the cycle at which the drug should be administered are questions which require further examination in the future.

# Double-blind crossover study of danazol versus placebo in the treatment of severe fibrocystic breast disease

A. GORINS, F. PERRET, B. TOURNANT, C. ROGIER AND J. LIPSZYC

*University of Paris VIIIᵉ, Hôpital Saint-Louis, Paris, France*

Danazol is an antigonadrotrophin, the therapeutic efficacy of which in endometriosis is well known. Several studies have also indicated that it constitutes a useful therapy for benign mammary dystrophy with a severe course (Aksu *et al.* 1978; Dhont *et al.* 1979; Gorins 1980; Mansel *et al.* 1982). In this paper, we report on the first French study in this field.

## Patients and methods (Fig. 1)

This study of danazol versus placebo was carried out under double-blind conditions. Each patient, acting as her own control, was allocated randomly to one or other of two groups. Patients in group 1 received two capsules daily of danazol ($2 \times 200$ mg) for three months followed by two capsules of placebo for a further three months. Patients in group 2 received danazol and placebo in reverse order. In all cases treatment started the day after menstruation.

Forty-five patients were involved in the study; all were premenopausal, their ages ranging from 28 to 55 years, with a mean of 42 years. In most cases the patients had previously received various forms of therapy (for example, anti-inflammatory agents, bromocriptine, synthetic progestational agents) with inadequate results, transient improvement or no improvement at all.

Results were assessed on the basis of changes in symptomatology (mastodynia, breast tension) and on improvement in clinical signs (modifications in the cysts, nodules and adenomatous areas). In addition, infra-red thermography was carried out before treatment during the last 15 days of treatment 'A' and during the last 15 days of treatment 'B', in order to assess changes in the overall heat of the breasts and the extent, richness and thickness of the vascular network.

Side effects were carefully monitored throughout the trial.

**Figures 4–9 in this paper are to be found in the colour section at the end of the symposia.**

*Benign Breast Disease, Edited by M. Baum, W. D. George, and L. E. Hughes, 1985: Royal Society of Medicine International Congress and Symposia series No. 76, published by the Royal Society of Medicine.*

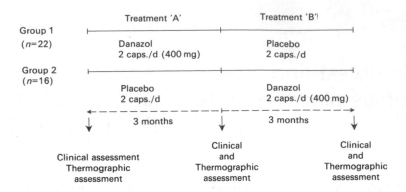

Fig. 1. *Danazol versus placebo: scheme of randomized double-blind crossover study.*

Of the 45 patients to whom the treatment was administered, seven dropped out and were eliminated from the study. Thus 38 patients (84 per cent) completed the trial.

## Results

### Clinical results

At the end of each therapeutic period, patients were assessed as clinically improved (objectively or subjectively), no change or worse, compared with the previous clinical examination. Thermographic results were similarly assessed. Because of the possibility of an order effect in the placebo period, the results of the two groups were analysed separately.

For patients in group 1 (Table 1) the clinical results were statistically in favour of danazol ($P < 0.001$). Of the 19 patients who improved on danazol, 10 maintained their improvement, either completely or partially, during the placebo period that followed.

For patients in group 2 (Table 2), the clinical results were also statistically in favour of danazol ($P < 0.05$).

The level of pain, as measured on a five-point rating scale, was reduced by danazol in group 1 patients and rose again on placebo (Fig. 2). When placebo was given first (group 2 patients) there was slight benefit, but in the danazol treatment period that followed there was a very clear decrease in pain (Fig. 3).

Table 1

*Clinical results (group 1),* n = 22

|  | Improved | No change | Worse |
|---|---|---|---|
| Danazol | 19* | 3 | 0 |
| Placebo | 0 | 10 | 12 |

*$P < 0.001$.

Table 2
Clinical results (group 2), n=16

|  | Improved | No change | Worse |
|---|---|---|---|
| Placebo | 7 | 8 | 1 |
| Danazol | 13* | 3 | 0 |

*P<0·05.

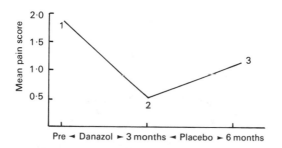

Fig. 2. Mean pain scores, both breasts (group 1), n=22.

## Thermographic results

For purposes of statistical analysis, patients who showed no change in their condition were considered together with those whose condition worsened. Because there was no possibility of order effect in the thermographic results, patients in groups 1 and 2 were evaluated as a whole.

Thermographic results for both groups are given in Table 3 and show that improvement on danazol was statistically significant ($P<0·001$).

Examples of thermographic results seen are shown in Figs 4–6 (group 1 patients) and in Figs 7–9 (group 2 patients).

## Side effects (Table 4)

Menstrual disturbance is almost a constant feature of danazol administration; of the 38 patients who completed this study, only three experienced no disturbance of menstruation. Weight gain was observed in 23 patients (60·5 per cent) and ranged from 1 kg to 7 kg over the treatment period of three months (mean 2·3 kg); the remaining 15 patients gained no weight at all. Other side effects occurred (vertigo, hot flushes) but these were less numerous and not considered to be significant. Side effects with placebo were also reported.

## Discussion

Danazol is clearly effective in the treatment of severe benign mastopathy and this study confirmed the results achieved by other workers, notably those of Dhont *et al.* (1979) and Mansel *et al.* (1982). Although the protocol of our trial was very similar to

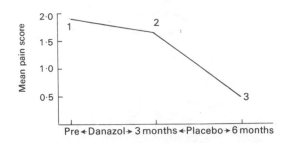

Fig. 3. Mean pain scores, both breasts (group 2), n=16.

Table 3

Thermographic results (groups 1 and 2), n=37

|  | Improved | No change or worse |
|---|---|---|
| Danazol | 28* | 9 |
| Placebo | 6 | 31 |

*$P < 0.01$.

Table 4

Side efects

|  | Danazol, *n* | Placebo, *n* |
|---|---|---|
| Menstrual disturbances | 30 | 5 |
| Weight gain | 23 (mean 2·3 kg) | 4 (mean 2 kg) |
| Arterial hypertension | 1 | 0 |
| Acne | 0 | 0 |
| Virilization | 1 (moderate) | 0 |
| Hot flushes | 4 | 2 |
| Other | Alopecia; heaviness of legs; vertigo; nausea | Headache; rash; gastric pain; nausea; dyspareunia |

that used by Mansel, it differed in two respects: we had a higher number of patients (our trial, 38 patients; Mansel, 22) and the use of infra-red thermography in our trial was an original note. Infra-red thermography is, of course, perfectly harmless and we find the technique extremely useful in following up patients with benign mastopathy. It cannot, however, be relied upon for the detection of breast cancer.

The dosage of danazol and the period of time for which it should be administered are still matters for further investigation. For benign breast disease the average dosage is said to be 400 mg per day, but Mansel *et al.* (1982) found that 200 mg danazol daily produced results approximately as good, although they took somewhat longer to achieve. Mansel and his collaborators found side effects at the 400 mg per day level too severe for their liking.

This is not an opinion we share. We make a practice of warning patients receiving danazol of the possibility of menstrual disturbance and of moderate weight gain and we recommend a low carbohydrate and low fat diet. Thus, in this study, no severe side effects were recorded and no patient discontinued treatment.

We propose at a later date to study the optimum dosage and duration of treatment of danazol, to compare the agent with synthetic progestational agents and to follow up the medium- and long-term progress of patients after discontinuation of hormone therapy.

## Summary

In this paper, we report a double-blind crossover study in which we compare the effects of danazol with placebo in 38 patients suffering severe benign mastopathy. The clinical and thermographic results were significantly in favour of danazol.

Thermography enabled us to add a very interesting and useful objective contribution to the evaluation of results.

Side effects were relatively common but moderate and did not prevent the continuation of treatment.

In the light of these results, it is concluded that danazol constitutes a powerful agent in the treatment of severe benign mastopathy.

## References

Aksu, M. F., *et al.* (1978). *J. Reprod. Med.,* **21**, 181–4.
Dhont, M., *et al.* (1979). *Postgrad. Med. J.,* **55** (Suppl. 5), 66–70.
Gorins, A. (1980). *Contraception–sexualité–fertilité,* **9**, 117–21.
Mansel, R. E., *et al.* (1982). *Lancet,* **i** (8278), 928–30.

# Results of the clinical evaluation of danazol in benign breast disease compared with local treatment, gestagens and bromocriptine

**R. GOEBEL**

*Evangelical Hospital, Oberhausen, West Germany*

It is a pleasure for me to participate in this symposium and to have the opportunity of presenting the results of these clinical studies on benign breast disease. The studies commenced in 1975 at the First Department of Obstetrics and Gynaecology of the University of Munich in Bavaria and continued at a women's hospital in the Ruhr area of West Germany.

## Materials and methods

In the eight years 1975–82, two randomized studies were carried out to evaluate the influence of medication on benign breast conditions in a total of 454 patients. The drugs used in both studies are shown in Table 1.

An anti-inflammatory isopropanol gel was used for local application. The second preparation was the phytotherapeutic agent Mastodynon, the main constituent of which is vitex agnus castus, which counteracts hyperfolliculinism by an effect similar to that of the corpus luteum. Mastodynon also contains plant extracts with spasmolytic and sedative properties.

Two gestagens were selected: a derivative of nortestosterone, norethisterone acetate, and a retroprogesterone, dydrogesterone. Bromocriptine and danazol were the other two agents used in the study.

Patients included in the study and treated with one or other of these six agents were suffering from either mastodynia (first series) or mastopathy (second series).

The term mastodynia was taken to mean unilateral or bilateral breast pain with painful swelling and a feeling of tension, together with a pronounced hyperalgesia of the nipple, the symptoms occurring cyclically and mainly in the luteal phase.

Two hundred and twelve women, whose main symptom was mastodynia, with no appreciable changes on mammography or on palpation, were randomized and treated according to one of the six therapy schedules (Table 1). About 70 per cent of these

*Benign Breast Disease, Edited by M. Baum, W. D. George, and L. E. Hughes, 1985: Royal Society of Medicine International Congress and Symposia series No. 76, published by the Royal Society of Medicine.*

Table 1

Therapy of benign breast disease: random studies 1975–82

| Therapy | Number of patients* | | Dosage per day |
|---|---|---|---|
| | Group 1 (n = 212) | Group 2 (n = 242) | |
| Local treatment (Hirudoid) | 37 | 40 | 2–4 g |
| Phytohormone (Mastodynon) | 41 | 42 | 3 × 20 drops |
| Norethisterone acetate | 34 | 43 | 10 mg (16th–25th days of cycle) |
| Dydrogesterone | 32 | 39 | 10 mg (16th–25th days of cycle) |
| Bromocriptine | 38 | 37 | 2·5 mg |
| Danazol | 33 | 41 | 200–400 mg |

*Group 1, mastodynia; group 2, mastopathy.

women complained also of symptoms of the premenstrual syndrome, but these were felt to be less irksome than the breast symptoms.

Patients were excluded from the studies if their brassieres were found to be poorly fitting, if they had orthopaedic abnormalities or if their breast symptoms were caused by hormonal disorders of other organs. Women with hyperprolactinaemia were also excluded (and treated primarily with bromocriptine).

Women in the second study group showed clinically and mammographically verified fibrocystic breast disease, with pain in one or both breasts, combined with tenderness and single or multiple nodules. Pain, tenderness and nodularity were evaluated during each therapeutic regimen; if a biopsy was indicated in a patient on the basis of mammographic and/or clinical examination, she was excluded from the study.

Two hundred and forty-two women, aged between 17 and 54 years, in this group were allocated to one of the treatment schedules in accordance with a treatment key previously laid down (Table 1).

The duration of the treatments was four to six months; dosages are set out in Table 1. Hirudoid was applied and massaged into the painful breast regions twice a day— about 2–4 g gel per application. Mastodynon was taken at a dosage of 3 × 20 drops per day. Norethisterone acetate and dydrogesterone were usually given for six months (10 mg per day from the 16th to the 25th day of the cycle). Women allocated to the bromocriptine group received 2·5 mg per day for four to six months. Women with mastodynia took 200 mg danazol per day and those with mastopathy, 400 mg danazol per day, in both cases for four to six months. Before, during and after treatment with danazol, the gonadotropins LH and FSH, prolactin, oestradiol-17β and progesterone were assayed. At each control investigation, LH- and FSH-stimulation tests were carried out.

All patients were recalled for control investigations at four-week intervals, at which time they filled in control forms for effects and side effects of the therapy. All women in the second investigation group (patients with mastopathy) were given control mammography at the end of the treatment.

## Results

Results of treatment with the various therapy schedules for patients with mastodynia are given Table 2. A positive effect of the treatment (freedom from or alleviation of symptoms) was achieved with the six different agents in 60–88 per cent of the women. However, there was a significant difference in freedom of symptoms between patients who received local treatment compared and those on systemic therapy.

In patients with mastodynia, no difference was found between Mastodynon, gestagens and bromocriptine in the rate of response of symptoms. The greatest number became free of symptoms on danazol, even though the difference compared with gestagen, bromocriptine and Mastodynon treatment had only low significance. Most women perceived marked improvement in their symptoms one to three months after the beginning of therapy. Usually, treatment for two to three months was necessary before patients became symptom-free. The results of each treatment for mastopathy patients are given in Tables 3–5. There are marked differences in the effectiveness of hormonal and non-hormonal preparations in reduction of pain (Table 3), reduction of breast tenderness (Table 4) and improvement in nodularity (Table 5).

*Table 2*
*Results of treatment in patients with mastodynia (group 1, n = 212)*

| Therapy | Complete relief (per cent) | Partial relief (per cent) | No relief (per cent) |
|---|---|---|---|
| Local treatment | 19 | 41 | 40 |
| Phytohormone | 49 | 22 | 29 |
| Norethisterone acetate | 47 | 35 | 18 |
| Dydrogesterone | 41 | 31 | 28 |
| Bromocriptine | 45 | 18 | 37 |
| Danazol | 58 | 30 | 12 |

*Table 3*
*Results of treatment in patients with mastopathy (breast pain) (group 2, n = 242)*

| Therapy | Complete relief (per cent) | Partial relief (per cent) | No relief (per cent) |
|---|---|---|---|
| Local treatment | 13 | 25 | 62 |
| Phytohormone | 43 | 17 | 40 |
| Norethisterone acetate | 49 | 23 | 28 |
| Dydrogesterone | 46 | 28 | 26 |
| Bromocriptine | 35 | 24 | 41 |
| Danazol | 51 | 27 | 22 |

Table 4

*Results of treatment in patients with mastopathy (breast tenderness) (group 2, n=242)*

| Therapy | Complete relief (per cent) | Partial relief (per cent) | No relief (per cent) |
|---|---|---|---|
| Local treatment | 18 | 38 | 44 |
| Phytohormone | 29 | 33 | 38 |
| Norethisterone acetate | 51 | 28 | 21 |
| Dydrogesterone | 44 | 33 | 23 |
| Bromocriptine | 41 | 30 | 29 |
| Danazol | 63 | 27 | 10 |

Table 5

*Results of treatment in patients with mastopathy (breast nodularity) (group 2, n=242)*

| Therapy | Complete regression (per cent) | Partial regression (per cent) | No regression (per cent) |
|---|---|---|---|
| Local treatment | 0 | 3 | 97 |
| Phytohormone | 5 | 14 | 81 |
| Norethisterone acetate | 21 | 28 | 51 |
| Dydrogesterone | 28 | 26 | 46 |
| Bromocriptine | 41 | 30 | 43 |
| Danazol | 66 | 22 | 12 |

Hirudoid alleviated breast pain and tenderness due to mastopathy, but not nodularity. Mastodynon had a similar effect (60 per cent of patients showed an alleviation of breast symptoms and tenderness of the breast) but reduction in size of fibrocystic nodules compared with initial findings was found only rarely on palpation or on control mammography at the end of therapy. On the other hand, treatment with both gestagens and the prolactin-inhibitor bromocriptine, gave freedom from symptoms or relief of breast pain as well as a favourable effect on nodularity in 60–80 per cent of the cases; however, gestagens and bromocriptine influenced fibrocystic nodularity only to a limited extent.

Danazol, though only slightly superior to other drugs in effectiveness against breast pain, was significantly better in its effect on nodularity of the breast (Table 5). With danazol, complete regression of the fibrocystic mastopathy was achieved in 66 per cent of the cases and complete or partial regression in almost 90 per cent.

This high success rate was not achieved in an earlier pilot study in women with mastopathy treated with danazol for only three months. At least four to six months of danazol therapy is evidently necessary to achieve this response rate, as reported by other authors.

Of the group 2 women (patients treated for mastopathy), 115 have so far been followed up, clinically and mammographically, for a period of two years after the completion of their treatment. The long-term results in these women of the effectiveness of treatment on breast nodularity are listed in Table 6. The superiority of danazol in the treatment of pronounced mastopathy is even more marked here compared with other substances tested. Whereas gestagen, bromocriptine and non-hormonal therapy show complete or partial regression in barely 30 per cent of women after two years, complete or partial response to danazol was maintained in 65–70 per cent of patients.

Unfortunately, in contrast to the high level of effectiveness of danazol, androgenic- and anabolic-related side effects occur in a high percentage of the patients. The side effects of the other drugs tested were insignificant and less often led to discontinuation of the therapy (Table 7).

## Conclusion

Danazol showed the highest success rate of the hormonal and non-hormonal drugs tested for treatment of mastodynia or mastopathy. Whereas the superiority of danazol compared with gestagens and bromocriptine in the treatment of mastodynia and breast pain due to mastopathy is not highly significant, the short-term and, above all, the long-term effectiveness of danazol treatment is more convincing in cases of breast tenderness and breast nodularity.

As the side effects of the non-hormonal, gestagen-containing and prolactin-inhibiting substances are fewer than with danazol, these drugs should be preferred in

*Table 6*

*Evaluation of breast nodularity in 115 patients with mastopathy two years after therapy\**

| Therapy | Complete regression (per cent) | Partial regression (per cent) |
|---|---|---|
| Local treatment | (0)  0 | (3)  5 |
| Phytohormone | (5)  2 | (14) 16 |
| Norethisterone acetate | (21) 12 | (28) 15 |
| Dydrogesterone | (28) 10 | (26) 20 |
| Bromocriptine | (41)  9 | (30) 22 |
| Danazol | (66) 52 | (22) 16 |

\* Figures in parentheses relate to results at the end of the treatment period—see Table 5.

*Table 7*

*Side effects*

| Therapy | Incidence of Side effects (per cent) |
|---|---|
| Local treatment | — |
| Phytohormone | 1·2 |
| Norethisterone acetate | 7·8 |
| Dydrogesterone | 7·0 |
| Bromocriptine | 14·7 |
| Danazol (200 mg) | 42·4 |
| Danazol (400 mg) | 53·6 |

mastodynia and mild forms of mastopathy. However, with pronounced pain, sensitivity and fibrocystic mastopathy danazol treatment for at least four months is highly indicated.

Finally, it should be mentioned that one woman became pregnant during treatment with danazol (200 mg per day), although an intra-uterine device was in position.

In another patient who received a gestagen preparation, a suspect mammary tumour was shown in the control mammogram carried out six months after the beginning of therapy. This proved to be a mammary carcinoma 0·7 cm in diameter.

# The management of breast pain in the Nottingham City Hospital Breast Pain Clinic

## C. P. HINTON

*City Hospital, Nottingham, England*

## Introduction

The Nottingham City Hospital is one of two teaching hospitals serving a population of about 750 000. Two-thirds of all women in the Nottingham area presenting with breast symptoms come to the Nottingham City Hospital Breast Clinic, which is under the direction of Professor R. W. Blamey. Between 1500 and 2000 new patients are seen in the breast clinic every year.

Breast pain is a very common symptom. Of the new patients presenting every year to the breast clinic, 20–25 per cent cite breast pain either as their only symptom or as one of their main symptoms. In the past, in many centres, breast pain has been considered important only as a possible sign of carcinoma, and in the absence of a lump or other signs of breast cancer no treatment has been offered. We feel that this attitude is not appropriate to the patient's needs and have set up a breast pain clinic to investigate these patients and to treat them when necessary.

## The classification of breast pain

Most patients presenting with breast pain require only reassurance, but a few require further investigation and treatment. The Nottingham Breast Pain Clinic was set up in 1978 and in the next four years 316 patients have been referred from the diagnostic clinic. These were those whose breast pain was considered to be sufficiently severe to warrant treatment. From our experience with these patients we have been able to classify patients with breast pain into three groups: (*a*) patients with true breast pain (70 per cent); (*b*) those with musculo-skeletal pain—most commonly due to cervical spondylosis or Tietze's syndrome (20–25 per cent); (*c*) a small group of other patients (5–10 per cent) with a variety of conditions, including cancer phobia, psychosexual problems and pregnancy presenting with breast pain. In most cases treatment follows logically from correct classification.

Of patients presenting with true breast pain, by far the largest number have cyclical breast pain. I will consider their management in detail. Typically, such patients experience a crescendo of pain rising towards the end of the menstrual cycle and ceasing at, or shortly after, the onset of menstruation (Fig. 1).

*Benign Breast Disease, Edited by M. Baum, W. D. George, and L. E. Hughes, 1985: Royal Society of Medicine International Congress and Symposia series No. 76, published by the Royal Society of Medicine.*

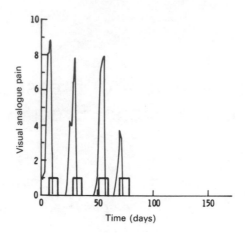

Fig. 1. Breast pain trial: cyclical breast pain. Curves indicate visual analogue pain; histograms indicate the occurrence of periods.

## The management of cyclical breast pain

When the pain clinic was established, many treatments for cyclical breast pain were advocated: two seemed to show particular promise—danazol and bromocriptine. We therefore embarked upon a clinical trial to assess these two agents and their relative efficacy. This was a double-blind, placebo-controlled trial in which 40 per cent of the patients received danazol, 100 mg t.d.s., 40 per cent bromocriptine, 2·5 mg b.d., and the remaining 20 per cent placebo. Three periods of assessment were involved: the two months preceding treatment (only paracetamol being allowed), a three-month treatment period during the administration of the trial drug, and by a two-month assessment period after treatment had been stopped.

As there is no biochemical or radiological test for cyclical breast pain, criteria for entry into the trial had to be on strict clinical grounds and recruitment has therefore been slow. To date, 39 patients have completed the trial and are available for assessment; preliminary results are worthy of consideration.

Figure 2 shows the results so far for danazol treatment compared with placebo. As the trial progressed a large number of placebo patients dropped out, leaving only a very small number receiving placebo towards the end of the trial. Danazol patients had rapid relief of their pain in the first two weeks of treatment whereas placebo patients were not relieved at all, and this was statistically significant ($P < 0.05$, Student's $t$ test). Compared with bromocriptine (Fig. 3), relief of pain with danazol was faster and better maintained. The differences between the groups being significant after two weeks ($P < 0.05$, $t$ test) and three months ($P < 0.05$) of treatment, and one month after treatment ($P < 0.02$). These preliminary results suggest that danazol is significantly more effective than either placebo or bromocriptine in the treatment of cyclical breast pain.

This finding mirrored our early results from an uncontrolled pilot study conducted in the breast pain clinic in which danazol provided relief in 11 out of 16 patients (69 per cent), compared with bromocriptine which provided relief in eight of 24 (33 per cent), and it was these results that led to our choosing danazol as our first-line treatment for patients outside the trial.

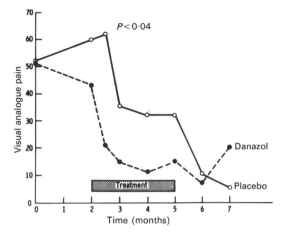

Fig. 2. Breast pain trial: danazol versus placebo.

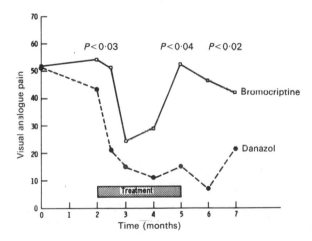

Fig. 3. Breast pain trial: danazol versus bromocriptine.

In the breast pain clinic we have seen 157 patients with cyclical breast pain severe enough to merit treatment. Of these, 97 were treated with danazol (100 mg t.d.s. for three months) and 83 are available for assessment having been followed up for at least six months. Seventy-one patients (86 per cent) responded with complete relief of pain or with sufficient relief to require only simple analgesia (paracetamol) to control it.

It is in the nature of the disease to relapse when treatment is stopped and indeed 32 per cent of patients did so. However, in over 80 per cent successful control of symptoms was achieved by a second or subsequent course of danazol.

Much has been made of the side effects of danazol, but we have found side effects to be a minor problem. Only nine of 97 patients have had side effects sufficiently severe to warrant withdrawal of treatment; it is interesting to note that four of the nine had complete relief of their pain prior to withdrawal of the drug and that these patients have not relapsed. We do not consider amenorrhoea a serious side effect; patients are warned that it may occur and most find it an advantage rather than a drawback.

Weight gain, although frequently occurring, has been modest in amount and has not led any patient to abandon treatment. The most important reason for treatment withdrawal was the onset of migrainous headaches, and this accounted for eight of the nine patients withdrawn from treatment. Some patients developed acne which settled after the end of treatment, and two patients developed mild ankle oedema which also disappeared when treatment was stopped.

## Conclusions

The vast majority of patients presenting at a breast clinic with cyclical breast pain of a mild nature require nothing more than reassurance that they do not have breast cancer. Only a small number will require treatment, and these may be managed with support and analgesics. In patients who fail to respond to these simple measures diuretics are occasionally helpful, but most will require more specific treatment. Our first-line treatment for severe cyclical breast pain is danazol. If danazol is contraindicated for any reason, bromocriptine remains a useful alternative.

Patients with severe cyclical breast pain can, in the majority of cases, be satisfactorily treated with danazol. Pain relief is achieved in 85 per cent of cases.

# Discussion: Session 4

**Baum**

I have a question for Dr Kruse. Just for clarification, you said the study comparing tamoxifen and danazol was a prospective study: was it a randomized trial?

**Kruse**

It was alternate treatment, not randomized.

**Baum**

There was another point I was not clear about. There were 350 cancers from 12 000 new attenders. Now that can't be a symptomatic clinic? Was it a screening clinic?

**Junkermann**

It is not just a symptomatic clinic. It is a screening clinic as well.

**Baum**

Thank you, that clarifies the point. It is a well-woman clinic and a symptomatic clinic also.

**Leinster**

Mr Kissin, it is not quite clear to me how you scored the changes in the mammographic pattern. Were these done blind? Can you comment on the reproducibility? You said it was done by two people; how comparable were their findings?

**Kissin**

The radiologist was a consultant radiologist, the clinician was myself. Agreement was generally good. Scoring was either 'no change', 'slight change' or 'marked change'. Agreement was quite good at both ends of this spectrum and less good in the middle, as you might expect.

**Leinster**

But did you ever feed yourself the same X-rays several times?

**Kissin**

Yes.

*Benign Breast Disease, Edited by M. Baum, W. D. George, and L. E. Hughes, 1985: Royal Society of Medicine International Congress and Symposia series No. 76, published by the Royal Society of Medicine.*

**Leinster**

I see, you did. But how good was the reproducibility?

**Kissin**

Reproducibility was good.

**Baum**

Was there a control group? Mammograms of patients who had no treatment?

**Kissin**

No, there was not. This wasn't a controlled trial. In another study it would be very interesting to see what happens with Panadol, a diuretic or no treatment at all.

**Perry**

No-one has mentioned the complications that I have had with danazol, severe muscle pain and cramp. I had one dear lady who had lockjaw and had to have her jaw unlocked by a dentist. Another lady had back pain which went on for 18 months. Maybe these patients had other problems, but they seemed to occur coincidentally with danazol treatment. The dose was a very low one. I'd like to know if anyone else has seen these problems.

**Potts**

Muscle cramps have been reported; that is a real adverse reaction. The incidence is small but we have seen it in our large-scale trials. The side effect is readily reversible. We have considered several possible sources of the problem, for example the potassium levels, but we've been unable to establish the cause of the muscle cramps.

**Gorins**

I have a question for Dr Kruse about tamoxifen. If I understood you correctly, you prescribed 10 mg per day, which is a low dosage. But in premenopausal women you have the problem of feedback mechanism, so is it not possible that you had a hypergonadrotropic effect with the anti-oestrogen, which induced a hyperoestrogeny which is undesirable?

**Junkermann**

May I answer the question? In this series of cases we did not measure the hormones. But we are now in the process of trying to find out what happens normally. With a low dosage of tamoxifen you go into the feedback mechanism. We know that in anovulatory women with tamoxifen we can induce ovulation by the feedback mechanism. But in our cases, clinically, we had menstrual irregularities in about 30 per cent with tamoxifen, about the same as with danazol, and we had some side effects of the hypo-oestrogenism type, but nothing indicative of hyperoestrogenism, no worsening, for example, of the breast disease in any of the cases.

**Gorins**

Another question, this time for Professor Goebel. Is it reasonable to compare continuous therapy with one agent with intermittent therapy with another agent?

**Goebel**

Well, that was the schedule which we chose. We chose this particular schedule because, in Germany, very often the gynaecologist uses this sort of schedule and administers gestagens cyclically. We know, of course, that results might be different if we gave gestagens through-out the cycle and perhaps that study is the next one we must do.

**Baum**

So, effectively, the trial was a pragmatic one. It was comparing what is done one way with what is done another way.

**Gorins**

My third question is for Mr Kissin. It concerns his justification for the hazards of repeated doses of radiation to the breast for xero-mammography.

**Kissin**

I agree that the dose of radiation is unacceptable if one is doing it in the repeated situation. The facilities were the only ones open to me. If onc is contemplating using something in the long term, then one can use xeromammography with techniques to reduce the dose, negative mode and so forth. But overall, in the context of a screening unit, if you're taking just two films, as compared with several films over a few years, the total radiation dose is not going to be a lot different.

**Baum**

Yes, but you take the point? We are talking about a cumulative dose of some significance.

**Kissin**

Oh yes. But as a one-off exercise to determine the effect, ethically I think this was acceptable.

**Parbhoo**

This is a question for Dr Kruse and her colleagues. I was fascinated by the report of the use of acupuncture in the treatment of benign breast disease and since this is cheap and highly effective in their hands, could they please elaborate on the method?

**Junkermann**

I didn't do the acupuncture myself; it was done by a colleague. But we were all very impressed by the high degree of pain relief which the patient reported. However, the problem seems to be that although there is a quick effect, the effect wears off. I think there is a strong element of suggestion involved and the technique cannot be placebo-controlled.

**Kumar**

I have two questions. The first is for Professor Shaikh. You made a comment that no patient was allowed a concomitant oral contraceptive. What was the reason? Is this not likely to lead to a greater morbidity?

**Shaikh**

After all, danazol does affect the hormonal levels. We stopped oral contraceptives for a month so that we could achieve a 'pure' effect, for the sake of simplicity, and because, frankly, we were not sure of what interactions there might be.

**Kumar**

My second question is for Mr Hinton. One of the features of double-blind trials is that the patient is unable to identify the agents. How do you double-blind danazol with bromocriptine?

**Hinton**

The protocol of the trial requires that patients take both sets of agents, one or both of which are a 'dummy'. They take them simultaneously and everyone appears to take both agents.

**Powley**

I'm a simple surgeon. In our part of the world, we've found that in carcinoma of the prostate you have to reduce the dose from 25 mg a day to 1 mg a day; so I decided to reduce the dose of danazol to 100 mg on alternate days. I found that we achieved the same sort of response rate that others were getting on the higher dose, and with fewer side effects in fact.

**Baum**

I think a number of speakers were getting round to addressing that issue. Professor Gorins was making the point that we're really not sure of the dosage and the scheduling. There is some clinical experience that needs pursuing.

**Preece**

I would like to put a question to both Mr Kissin and Professor Shaikh. Both mentioned that the patients they were treating demonstrated a reduction in breast size. Could I ask each of them to tell us how they measured that?

**Shaikh**

One of the patients had fibroadenosis, painful nodularity in one breast, and that was her main complaint. She herself said that her breast was getting bigger. On inspection it was indeed bigger than the other breast. After danazol treatment, the breast was noticeably smaller in size and both breasts became more or less equal. Also, the nodularity had disappeared from the affected breast along with the pain. The same sort of thing occurred in another patient. So it was not really a matter of measuring the breast-size reduction. Although we did relatively few mammograms, reduction in breast size was seen there also.

**Kissin**

Our conclusions were entirely subjective and obviously not scientific, but we were dealing with a small number of patients whom we were seeing regularly. However, at the end of treatment when the breast is smaller, it is often quite floppy and loose in some patients, because it's lost its nodularity. And some patients don't like it because you've given them a postmenopausal breast prematurely.

**Rickett**

Can I take up a point that was made about unmasking of breast cancer? Danazol has in fact been used in the treatment of advanced breast cancer and it may cause regression of a small primary tumour. This is obviously significant and I wondered whether anyone would like to comment on it.

**Baum**

That is a nice point. What you are suggesting is that it may clean out the mammogram and at the same time diminish the size of the cancer so that we miss it altogether. Mr Kissin you raised this. Would you care to comment?

**Kissin**

I didn't want to be too controversial and claim that danazol might produce regression. It would be useful enough if danazol were to reveal something that was there, but really nice if it could produce tumour regression as well.

**Baum**

It does certainly have some biological effect on some breast cancers.

**Herrmann**

Almost the same question. Nowadays, worldwide, many thousands of women have been treated with danazol, many of them for so-called mastopathy, these being patients at risk of getting breast cancer. Is there anything known about the breast cancer rate in these treated patients? And apart from the clinical and mammographic evidence that we've heard discussed, are there any data on histological response? Naturally, we want to treat the disease and not just the symptom.

**Baum**

That's a very difficult question. I doubt if anyone in the audience has the answer. But it might be an appropriate question to end the meeting on, because really you have just suggested the next 10 years of research with danazol. I think to answer the question would demand some very large-scale epidemiological studies, perhaps randomized, to see the long-term effects of this obviously very potent agent on the incidence of benign pathology, premalignant pathology and cancer itself.

# Session 4:

## CHAIRMAN'S SUMMARY

### M. BAUM

*King's College Hospital Medical School,*
*London, England*

Undoubtedly, danazol has a clinical effect in patients with painful breasts, lumpy breasts and painful, lumpy breasts. This, if nothing else, may allow us to have some insight into the mechanisms behind the aetiology of this disease. Perhaps danazol has a research role in dissecting out the mechanisms of the disease.

As far as its clinical role is concerned, I think it is quite clear from what all the speakers have said, and nicely summarized in the paper from Nottingham at the end of the session, that there is a place for danazol in a strategy of treating painful, lumpy breasts. Certainly exclude those patients who have cancer phobia; certainly postpone a decision to give treatment until the symptoms persist in spite of strong reassurance. You are then left with a sub-group of women in whom the symptoms themselves are worse than the possible side effects.

What I have found interesting this afternoon in the papers presented on danazol is the contrast between the percentage of side effects reported and the seriousness of those side effects. What came out was that the side effects appeared to be more prominent in those studies where there was no placebo control group. It is obvious that in this type of disease, placebo-controlled trials are important, not only to demonstrate the therapeutic benefit but also to demonstrate that the placebo itself has side effects.

I think it is quite clear, therefore, that there is a minority of patients, who can be identified, for whom treatment with danazol is of undoubted benefit and more than compensates for the somewhat minimal side effects. You can always stop the treatment when there are migrainous headaches; you can warn the patients about the incidence of amenorrhoea; and remember that, in any case, the side effects are reversible.

We have a lot more to learn about the disease and its treatment and the natural history of benign disease has to be elucidated.

But as far as therapeutic strategies are concerned we still need to know a lot more about the appropriate dose-scheduling of danazol and the duration of response. I, for one, use the drug frequently, but I don't know how long to give it for, when to stop and, on stopping, when to restart it if necessary. I think there is more than enough room for work to be done to warrant a further meeting of this type.

*Benign Breast Disease, Edited by M. Baum, W. D. George, and L. E. Hughes, 1985: Royal Society of Medicine International Congress and Symposia series No. 76, published by the Royal Society of Medicine.*

# Session 5:
# The Hjørring project

## CHAIRMAN'S INTRODUCTION

### W. D. GEORGE

*University of Glasgow and Western Infirmary,*
*Glasgow, Scotland*

Hjørring, in case you are wondering, is in Denmark in the north of Jutland. The project that began there three-and-a-half years ago is based on a breast clinic that was started in 1965 by Dr Rasmussen. This clinic has followed up a large number of patients over many years and so has a very good data base of patients about whom many factors are known and upon whom this project was centred.

The principal aim of the project was to examine the clinical, endocrine and mammographic aspects of benign breast disease and to see how these might be altered by treatment with danazol.

*Benign Breast Disease, Edited by M. Baum, W. D. George, and L. E. Hughes, 1985: Royal Society of Medicine International Congress and Symposia series No. 76, published by the Royal Society of Medicine.*

# The Hjørring project on fibrocystic breast disease*

## TH. RASMUSSEN,[1] A. DOBERL,[3] G. RANNEVIK[2] AND T. TOBIASSEN[2]

[1]*Department of Radiodiagnostics and* [2]*Department of Obstetrics and Gynaecology, Hjørring County Hospital, Hjørring, Denmark,* [3]*Deparmtnet of Clinical Research, Sterling-Winthrop Scandinavia, Solna, Sweden, and Fertility Research Institute, Malmo, Sweden*

## Patient selection criteria and definition of the clinical material

Two types of patient with benign breast disease have presented particular problems: first, patients with severe mastalgia/mastodynia and, secondly, patients with chronic formation of macrocysts. Severe mastodynia lasting from one to three weeks per menstrual cycle is highly unpleasant and often impairs patients' physical and social function. Patients with chronic formation of macrocysts are a sizeable group—the majority produce several cysts per annum over a considerable number of years. Surgical removal of cysts is cosmetically unsatisfactory while puncture with aspiration and cytology of the aspirate is mere symptomatic treatment.

Patients were selected for danazol treatment on the basis of strict criteria regarding intensity and duration of mastodynia as well as palpatory and mammographic findings. All patients had pronounced and usually chronic symptoms. A total of 109 patients completed treatment. Their mean age was $40.0 \pm 6.2$ (s.d.) years (range 22–52). Forty-four per cent had a history of more than 10 years. The following variables were recorded and scored subjectively: mastodynia; mass of palpable structure; nodularity/isolated lumps; mammographic; adenosis; cysts (small, i.e. up to 1 cm; large, i.e. more than 1 cm); and finally ductectasia.

Before treatment, we made a particular effort to ensure correct diagnosis of each palpable nodularity and isolated lump during mammographic evaluation. Cysts of more than 1 cm were aspirated. Fibroadenomata were supplemented with adenography. Other lumps were visualized by means of galactography. As a result of these procedures, our 109 patients were classified into three diagnostic sub-groups: fibroadenosis without cysts ($n = 20$), mean ages.d. $33.1 \pm 5.5$ years; fibroadenosis + small cysts ($n = 43$), $39.2 \pm 4.9$ years; fibroadenosis + large cysts ($n = 46$), $43.7 \pm 4.6$ years.

---

* This article is a summary of papers actually presented at the symposium.

*Benign Breast Disease, Edited by M. Baum, W. D. George, and L. E. Hughes, 1985: Royal Society of Medicine International Congress and Symposia series No. 76, published by the Royal Society of Medicine.*

# Hormone patterns in patients with fibrocystic disease

In a previous communication (Rannevik *et al.* 1983) we reported elevated levels of sex hormone-binding globulin (SHBG) in patients with fibrocystic breast disease (FBD). SHBG levels are considered to reflect the influence of the androgen/oestrogen balance on protein synthesis in the liver. To investigate further the endocrine situation in the FBD patient, we have determined peripheral levels of androgens and of some steroid-sensitive proteins in FBD patients and in strictly age-matched controls.

## Method
Plasma levels of dehydroepiandrosterone (DHA) and its sulphate (DHAS), androstenedione (A4), testosterone (T), SHBG, corticosteroid-binding globulin (CBG) and thyroxin-binding globulin (TBG) were determined in 54 normally menstruating FBD patients, aged $38 \cdot 8 \pm 5 \cdot 4$ ($m \pm$ s.e.m.) years and in 27 age-matched healthy controls aged $39 \cdot 0 \pm 5 \cdot 4$ years. Patients and controls were almost identical with respect to body weight ($59 \cdot 5 \pm 7 \cdot 6$ versus $60 \cdot 0 \pm 8 \cdot 2$ kg) and to Brocas' index ($0 \cdot 94 \pm 0 \cdot 13$ versus $0 \cdot 95 \pm 0 \cdot 14$).

## Results
Significantly higher values were found in FBD patients compared with controls for DHA ($P < 0 \cdot 02$), DHAS ($P < 0 \cdot 01$), A4, SHBG, CBG and TBG ($P < 0 \cdot 001$ for each). T levels were slightly, but not significantly, elevated in FBD patients.

## Conclusions
The unexpected combination of elevated androgen- and steroid-sensitive protein values suggests a complex relationship between ovaries, liver, pituitary and adrenal cortex. The exact nature of these interactions is unknown. Possible mechanisms may involve an increased follicular steroid synthesis (A4, oestrogens), affecting liver metabolism and protein synthesis. The increased adrenocortical steroid synthesis (DHA, DHAS and part of A4) may be secondary to these effects.

# Results of primary treatment with danazol

Out of 109 patients treated with danazol for six months, 55 patients received 400 mg a day (200 mg b.d.) and 54 patients 200 mg a day (100 mg b.d.). There was no difference in age between the two groups (mean ages $\pm$ s.d., $40 \cdot 1 \pm 6 \cdot 4$ and $39 \cdot 9 \pm 6 \cdot 0$ years, respectively). Mastodynia responded rapidly and equally well to both doses. After one month, the mean intensity of mastodynia was reduced to mild, and after six months' treatment 90 per cent were completely free of mastodynia. The mass of palpable structure decreased dramatically in most cases; the breasts became softer and 'less filled'. Mammographically, adenosis was observed to decrease very significantly. Fibroadenomata decreased but did not disappear. Lumps of localized fibroadenosis gradually resolved and disappeared completely in two-thirds of patients. The mammographic appearance of small cysts and of the ductal system is deceptive. At first visualization increased due to regression of adenosis, i.e. cysts and ducts become less obscured by dense glandular tissue; thereafter they become less prominent due to decreased secretion.

Macrocysts: in 46 patients, before they entered the trial, 786 cysts were aspirated over a mean period of $3 \cdot 7$ years (mean, 107 aspirated cysts per six-month period during the years preceding the trial). Before treatment, and at three and six months of treatment, a further 98, 101 and 36 cysts, respectively, became accessible for puncture.

In contrast, during the first four six-month periods post-treatment, only one, three, seven and two cysts were punctured, i.e. a total of 13 cysts in two years post-treatment. In fact, only nine of 46 patients have so far relapsed with cysts, and even in these nine patients, the rate of cyst formation was less than half that of the years before treatment.

Thus, danazol not only offers effective symptomatic treatment, but also stops the development of large cysts for a considerable period after treatment.

## Time and rate of symptomatic relapse

The hormonal and metabolic actions of danazol are reversible, and so cyclical hormonal stimulation of target tissues, including those of the breast, resumes shortly after treatment. Therefore it was to be expected that symptoms would recur at some time after treatment, unless the patient reached the menopause.

In order to study how long patients may still benefit after a six-months' course of danazol treatment, all patients were re-examined three months after completed treatment and thereafter at six-month intervals for up to three years.

Relapse was defined as the time by which mastodynia had reached the same, or very nearly the same, intensity as before treatment. The results obtained so far reveal a trend towards a shorter mean interval to relapse, as well as a higher cumulative relapse rate in patients who had been treated originally with 200 mg a day for six months compared with those who had received 400 mg a day for six months (Table 1).

Table 1

Times and rates of symptomatic relapse

| Dosage | Mean interval to relapse | Cumulative relapse rate | Mean follow-up period |
|--------|--------------------------|-------------------------|------------------------|
| 200 mg | 9·2 months | 64 per cent | 18·2 months |
| 400 mg | 12·2 months | 50 per cent | 25·9 months |

At 12 months after treatment this difference in cumulative relapse rate was statistically significant. Moreover, since the mean post-treatment observation period was significantly longer in the 400 mg group than in the 200 mg group, the difference may become accentuated further as the post-treatment surveillance continues. This may be indicative of a more profound, and therefore perhaps more sustained, inactivation of the glandular tissue by the 400 mg a day dose.

There were no statistical differences with regard to age, pre-treatment clinical, mammographic or biochemical characteristics, or response to initial treatment between patients who relapsed and those who have not relapsed so far.

## Double-blind placebo-controlled treatment of symptomatic relapse

Patients with symptomatic relapse were entered in a double-blind, placebo-controlled, between-patient study. As 400 and 200 mg a day had produced equivalent clinical response in the open trial, the efficacy of a lower dose was evaluated in the double-blind study. Moreover, this study permitted a comparison of the response under double-blind conditions with the response of the same patients in the original open trial.

### Design

Fifteen patients each received either danazol or placebo in randomized fashion. During the first month, two capsules a day (danazol 100 mg or placebo) were given; thereafter, one capsule a day. If at the end of three months a patient had not experienced any relief of mastodynia and was unwilling to continue, the code was broken. Other patients continued medication at one capsule a day for a further three months.

### Results

In contrast to placebo, danazol caused a highly statistically significant reduction of the score for mastodynia. The difference between placebo and danazol was statistically significant at all times (one, three and six months). The superiority of danazol over placebo was equally significant with regard to the proportion of patients experiencing partial or complete relief of symptoms as well as the number of code-breaks due to lack of symptomatic relief.

The response to danazol in the double-blind study was remarkably similar to the response in the original open trial, demonstrating good reproducibility of results. However, 100 mg a day failed to produce a further decrease in mean score (mastodynia) between three and six months, the difference between 100 mg a day and the higher doses (200 or 400 mg a day) being statistically significant at six months. This suggests that, in severe cases, 100 mg a day may not be as effective as 200 or 400 mg a day in giving complete relief of symptoms.

## Conclusions

The Hjørring project attempted to answer several questions, and although some issues call for further investigations, the results obtained so far may be summarized as follows:

The increased serum levels of various hormones, basically oestrogen precursors, and of some steroid-sensitive plasma proteins, found in patients with severe symptomatic fibrocystic breast disease, strongly support the concept that biological hyper-oestrogenicity—albeit of unknown aetiology—plays a significant role in the development of this condition.

The efficacy of danazol as a treatment has been confirmed. Almost all patients responded with total or near-total elimination of symptoms, a marked reduction in heaviness of palpable structure, significant reduction in adenosis, softening and gradual resolution of isolated lumps, and arrested formation of large cysts. All these findings appear to be a consequence of the regression of glandular tissue, which has been documented mammographically.

In the majority of cases the therapeutic effect lasts for a considerable time after treatment. As expected, mastodynia may recur, but the mean interval to relapse is in the order of at least nine to 12 months. One-third of the patients in the 200 mg group, and half the patients in the 400 mg group, have not been in need of renewed treatment within an observation period of 18 months to two years. Of particular interest is the highly significant reduction in cyst formation several years after treatment.

Treatment of relapse under double-blind conditions confirmed the superiority of danazol over placebo as well as the reproducibility of the results of the open trial.

Doses of 100, 200 and 400 mg of danazol a day, given for six months, have been shown to be active. However, 100 mg a day may be somewhat less effective in eliminating symptoms in severe cases, and symptomatic relapses may occur sooner and more frequently after treatment with 200 mg instead of 400 mg a day.

## Reference

Rannevik, G., *et al.* (1983). In *Endocrinology of cystic breast disease* (ed. A. Angeli *et al.*), pp. 127–33. Raven Press, New York.

# Discussion: Session 5

**Gorins**

Has a correlation been found between the decrease in SHBG levels in patients on danazol and the clinical results obtained?

**Rannevik**

We have a direct method of assay for SHBG with very low inter- and intra-assay variation and the difference between the patients and normal females was highly significant. We didn't study post-menopausal women since the study was directed towards fibrocystic breast disease.

**Junkermann**

Dr Rannevik said that higher SHBG levels were found and that these were elevated by high oestrogen levels. Was free oestradiol measured in the samples? That would be very interesting because the differences in fibrocystic breast disease between the total oestradiol are not very profound; there are only small differences for a few days of the cycle and so it would be interesting to know whether free oestradiol was elevated.

**Rannevik**

I agree that it would be very interesting but we didn't do the measurement. But the SHBG levels may not be high, because of the elevated oestradiol, as we proposed; possibly we have genetically high SHBG levels in these patients.

**Junkermann**

If in these patients you have genetically high SHBG levels, then the oestradiol should be more bound and the tissues should be less oestrogenized.

**Rannevik**

Yes, but you will have even lower levels of free androgens so the oestradiol will be balanced.

**Gorins**

Do you agree that SHBG may enter into the cell by a membrane effect?

*Benign Breast Disease, Edited by M. Baum, W. D. George, and L. E. Hughes, 1985: Royal Society of Medicine International Congress and Symposia series No. 76, published by the Royal Society of Medicine.*

**Rannevik**

Nobody yet knows whether SHBG enters the cells.

**George**

Dr Rannevik, may I ask you to say something about the controls that you used, how you took the samples and at what stage in the cycle?

**Rannevik**

The controls were of the same age as the patients and mammographically normal.

**Rasmussen**

Yes, they were all clinically and mammographically normal with no sign of fibrocystic disease.

**Rannevik**

Also, there was no difference between the two groups in terms of the stage of the menstrual cycle at which samples were taken. Women in both groups were sampled once in the follicular phase and once in the luteal phase.

**Leinster**

Can I ask Dr Rasmussen what steps were taken to ensure that the exposure on mammography was the same on each occasion? Because it seems to me that if the breast is getting smaller on danazol treatment, as we've heard, to use the same X-ray exposure may actually result in an increased penetration which is going to complicate any comparison between the views.

**Rasmussen**

You are quite right. We have an automatic mammography device which reduces the dose and the exposure automatically.

**George**

As a corollary to that question, I notice that some of your patients were having seven or eight mammograms done over a period of about three years. Is that right?

**Rasmussen**

Yes.

**George**

Are you not concerned about that in terms of dosage?

**Rasmussen**

No, these patients had severe symptoms and we use very low dose mammography. I know it would be unwise to do it for a large number of years for all our patients but our experience and results help us to use the technique appropriately.

**Parbhoo**

My question is similar to that of Professor George. How do you justify the use of seven mammograms to the ethical committee?

**Rasmussen**

I have answered that question.

**Parbhoo**

Another question. Because the breasts are very tender and enlarged, when you use a compression technique do you have any difficulty as the breast becomes smaller?

**Rasmussen**

We do use a compression technique but because we use automatic mammography equipment which changes the exposure automatically, when we compress a little more because the breast is smaller, there is no change in the picture.

**Parbhoo**

I see, thank you.

**Shaikh**

I am getting the impression that good results are achieved with danazol in cystic disease when there are multiple cysts. The types of patients we have been treating were those with fibroadenosis with mastodynia where the cyst formation was not predominant. My impression has been that the patients with cyst formation are the more elderly ones who do not complain of pain so much. My point is that these are two different types of patients, with two different disease patterns; just as Mr Preece said yesterday, in the younger age-group there is fibroadenosis with pain without prominent cystic disease, whilst cyst formation is seen in the premenopausal older woman. How much pain did Dr Rasmussen's cystic disease patients have?

**Rasmussen**

They had just the same sort of pain or more. Sometimes it was impossible to palpate to find the cyst because of pain. We think that while patients with small cystic fibroadenosis are younger than those with large cysts, we may well meet the patient who now has microcysts 10 years hence with macrocysts.

**Hinton**

In talking about the characterization of the patients, one of the speakers showed that the group having 400 mg danazol included a larger number of patients who had their symptoms for more than 10 years, had a higher incidence of nodularity and more symptoms at the start of treatment. I would like to ask Dr Doberl if he thinks this relates to their increased relapse rate?

**Doberl**

On the contrary, patients receiving 400 mg danazol a day had a lower relapse rate.

**Hinton**

No, I'm sorry, that's not what I am asking. The point is that the groups are different and is it therefore valid to compare relapse rates in two groups who are different symptomatically at the start of treatment?

**Doberl**

We felt it was justified to do so because we had not found any significant difference in response in any variable we looked at during initial treatment. We found no difference in initial response between patients on 200 mg and those on 400 mg and, when we looked at the different types of patients, again we found no differences. Whatever parameter was looked at there were decreasing parallel curves. However, we have also looked at those patients who relapsed late to see if they were over-represented compared with those who relapsed early, and the answer was no. Also at patients with a particularly intense adenosis, or particularly lumpy breasts, to see if they were over-represented in those who relapsed early, but they were not. Neither was SHBG related to relapse. We looked at all these things but found no differences.

**George**

And did the mammograms change back to what they were originally on relapse?

**Doberl**

Yes. Dr Rasmussen will correct me if I'm wrong, but yes, the heaviness of palpable structures increases again and also the adenosis as visible on the mammogram does increase again.

**George**

And yet the cysts don't seem to come back?

**Doberl**

No, not so far.

**Gorins**

My feeling is that the majority of patients treated with danazol continue to benefit several months after treatment, sometimes for as long as a year or more. Would it not be reasonable to stop the treatment after three or six months and to resume treatment when there is relapse?

About the relapse: you study only the breasts, but I believe it is very important to consider the environment and the patient's psychological problems also. If you question your patients you often learn that the cysts appear after emotional crises. This information is very important and if the questions are asked you may find that emotional crises have occurred three times out of four, such as an illness in the family, problems with the children, or with the husband. With this in mind, we consider our patients' emotional problems in conjunction with a clinical psychologist.

**Doberl**

I must say that I was unaware of any correlation between the occurrence of a cyst and emotional stress and problems. Perhaps Dr Rasmussen would like to comment?

**Rasmussen**

I have heard you express this view once before, Professor Gorins. But I personally have never found any correlation between psychological problems and cysts. Patients seem to find them appearing quite suddenly, it is true, and they are very anxious when they find them, but whenever I have asked about emotional crises I have been unable to find out anything that would relate.

**Gorins**

And yet in my experience the correlation is very frequent.

**Porritt**

May I ask a very simple question? When patients relapse, are they so impressed with the danazol treatment they had earlier that they ask for further treatment or do you have to persuade them?

**Doberl**

Patients by no means need to be persuaded to accept re-treatment; they actually ask for it. All the patients in this study who relapsed, except for two, have started on a second course of treatment. The two exceptions have not yet started on a second course.

**Lloyd-Williams**

I have a fairly pragmatic approach to the matter of dosage and when patients have pain in the breast I have tended to give them hormones and say: 'take as much as you need'. The question, then, that I want to ask is, has anybody found out what lower level of danazol you can go down to? I have two patients who have been on 25 mg of danazol for six days before their period and they have adjusted this dosage themselves. The way I do it is to start off on 100 mg danazol a day and if they are comfortable on that but not pain-free, I tell them to try to cut down the dosage, to perhaps 50 mg a day or 100 mg every other day, to see if they are better on that dosage. Has anyone got any statistical data on really low maintenance dosage?

**Tobiassen**

We have not used dosages lower than 100 mg. In our series it became obvious that that was too low a dose and we would now not go lower than 200 mg.

**George**

That is an interesting question that has been raised before. I suggest we come back to it in the general discussion at the end of the symposium.

**Mansel**

Can you please explain how the mastodynia changes were assessed and by whom and what statistical tests were applied to find the *P*-values?

**Doberl**

Assessments were made by Dr Tobiassen and Dr Rasmussen according to a scoring system—pain, out of 1, 2 or 3, and other elements, 1, 2, 3 or 4. Mastodynia was assessed on the basis of examination and patient interview. The statistics applied were Willcoxon's tests, paired for observation, changes within the patient and between groups, between the placebo group and the danazol group.

**Benson**

Could I ask Dr Rasmussen, in view of the fact that there is undoubtedly a placebo effect, and you have shown it in the Hjørring project, do you get mammographic changes in patients who improve on placebo in the same way as you get mammographic improvement in the women who respond to the active agent?

**Rasmussen**

When we did do mammography, there were no clear signs of improvement on placebo that could compare with the effects of danazol. But mammography was not employed on all patients.

**Benson**

So there was symptomatic improvement not shown on mammography?

**Rasmussen**

Symptomatic and palpable improvement, yes.

**Preece**

As it was my brief to talk earlier in this symposium on nomenclature, I would like to discuss with Dr Rasmussen his use of the word 'heaviness' in relation to palpated structures. My understanding of the word, as he uses it, is that it meant the 'density' of the breast. Would Dr Rasmussen please clarify the point? Does he mean that the breast tissue is more dense to palpation?

**Rasmussen**

In my view, the term 'dense' is applied to what is seen in the mammogram; I cannot use the same term to describe what I see in the mammogram and what I feel in the breast, so I have to choose another word. I cannot describe precisely what it is I would score 4 for in heaviness, but with much experience in the palpation of the breast, one comes across a feeling of heaviness which is unmistakable to the single observer.

**Preece**

I think the 'single observer' component is very important here and I would support it from my own experience. However, I would like to suggest that we should try to find an alternative word to 'heaviness', because this word—at any rate in English-speaking countries—is one which the patient frequently volunteers for a symptom that they feel in their breast and, as we saw in Mr Mansel's visual analogue, this is one symptom which can be very precisely measured in terms of what the patient actually says. I am concerned that we might lose some clarity here, although I see your objection to 'density'. I wonder if anyone here can suggest a word which might have international acceptability.

**Doberl**

May I explain that Dr Rasmussen, in fact, uses a Danish word to describe what he feels, which translated literally means 'mass-feeling'. This sounds rather odd in English and we spent a lot of time in discussing an appropriate English term; obviously the one we chose is not the most appropriate one because you picked on it straight away.

**Walsh**

I have a question for Dr Rannevik. The oestrogens remained in normal concentration during treatment with either 200 or 400 mg danazol; can you tell me what happened to the progesterone concentration?

**Rannevik**

During the administration of 600 mg, there was no increase in progesterone concentrations in any patients. We have not yet analysed the figures for progesterone levels in patients on lower dosages; even if we were to find lowered progesterone concentrations, we would be unable to say that ovulation did not occur some time between taking samples.

**Baum**

Dr Rasmussen proposes a hypothesis that fibroadenosis proceeds to fibroadenosis plus microcysts which then proceeds, as part of a continuum, to fibroadenosis, microcysts and macrocysts. And yet the breast with pain and nodularity, following treatment with danazol, relapses in 50–60 per cent of cases, although almost none of the patients with macrocystic disease, multiple punctures, relapse on danazol. Surely that falsifies the hypothesis and one has to look again at two diseases rather than think of a continuum of one disease?

**Rasmussen**

As you said in your paper, Professor Baum, there are patients who have one cyst and never have another; that is quite another disease and not the one we are talking about. We have thought a lot about the mechanism of small cysts and large cysts. If you see small cysts filled galactographically and take a picture, 14 days or a month later you find they have emptied. If you have a patient with larger cysts, half a centimetre, one centimetre, and so on, and fill them galactographically, you can find the contrast medium still there a half-year after the injection. There is obviously some difference in the mechanism of filling and emptying between the small and the large cysts. Remember, we have had our clinic for 17 years; we have patients whose examinations have been two or three years apart and we have seen the development from a few, small cysts, hardly to be seen, to an overall cystic appearance and then, in some of them, large cysts, over a period of, I think, 12 years.

**George**

I think at this point we should bring this session to a close. I do not propose to reiterate all that has been said but I think this has been a very interesting session and the study a very good one, one in which the participants have tried extremely hard to record as much data as possible and to give us as full a presentation as possible. I am sure it has stimulated a number of thoughts that we can return to in the general discussion that follows.

# Session 6:
# Benign breast disease: whither the management?
# (general discussion)

## CHAIRMAN'S INTRODUCTION

### W. D. GEORGE

*University of Glasgow and Western Infirmary,*
*Glasgow, Scotland*

I think it would be useful to have a definition of the type of benign breast disease we are talking about. I don't think we are talking about cysts or fibroadenomas or other discreet lesions because we have all agreed that cysts should be aspirated and fibroadenomas removed.

What we are really talking about, therefore, is the problem of nodularity and pain; and certainly in the series presented by Professor Baum, about half the patients who presented with benign breast disease had pain and nodularity.

I think there are still arguments about this in terms of definition and whether this is really just a variant of normal; it is such a common symptom that it could almost be regarded as such. You might wish to comment on this and I think a brief discussion on definitions would be worthwhile. No doubt Mr Preece will have something to say.

I think, too, that there should be some discussion on the endocrine profiles in patients with benign breast disease, because if consistent changes are being shown we might be getting nearer to the mechanism of the abnormality.

One thing that has emerged from this meeting is that the figures presented by Mauvais-Jarvis cannot be substantiated by any other group and that, in a way, is quite a relief because otherwise a lot of people might be chasing lots of things for a long time.

It is interesting that the Scandinavian team has raised the SHBG story, which I suspect will have to be followed up by various groups.

One thing I am not entirely clear about is what is actually happening to oestradiol and progesterone levels in patients treated with danazol. From what we've heard it seems that nobody has yet described clearly what is happening in relationship to dose. We are told that on lower doses patients may well be ovulating but we have no clear information; Dr Potts might wish to comment and I know that Mr Mansel has some questions on the subject.

*Benign Breast Disease, Edited by M. Baum, W. D. George, and L. E. Hughes, 1985: Royal Society of Medicine International Congress and Symposia series No. 76, published by the Royal Society of Medicine.*

Certainly we have to address the question of low dosages: whether or not the effects of danazol at low doses are mediated at the pituitary or whether these effects are being mediated by changes in the blocking of receptors. Clearly, if the lower doses are working by the blocking of receptors, one might avoid a lot of the side-effect problems associated with the drug. So low dosage is a subject worth talking about. Also, I think we should talk about the place of different treatment modalities with painful, lumpy benign breast disease. Mr Hinton pointed out that the majority of women who present with these symptoms are treated adequately by reassurance or by simple analgesics and relatively few women progress to more complicated treatment.

We have a number of different treatments available: we can, for example, use diuretics, although most people would agree with Mr Hinton that diuretics are not very effective, but we also have progestogens and bromocriptine, and the former have fewer side effects than either bromocriptine or danazol; and we have danazol. So we should perhaps discuss the place of these different agents in the treatment of benign breast disease and how they should be used in some sort of logical sequence.

Lastly, perhaps we can find time to discuss the point raised by Professor Baum, how we can cut the cost to the patient and the cost to the health services, and here there is a relationship with how patients are managed on their first visit to the clinic. It would be interesting to have some comments on the role of aspiration cytology in these patients and the role of mammography.

Professor Baum has cast some doubts on the role of mammography. The Dundee group has perhaps had the most experience of these three modalities in conjunction, and so Mr Preece might like to comment.

Those are the broad areas we might discuss: what is normal and is not? What about the dosages of the drugs? How should we use them and in what order? How should we manage patients at the first clinic attendance?

I now open the session for general discussion.

# General discussion

## CHAIRMAN: W. D. GEORGE

*University of Glasgow and Western Infirmary,*
*Glasgow, Scotland*

---

### Benson

May I start off by making the point that if we take away fibrocystic disease and fibroadenoma, as the Chairman indicated, we are left with the problem of breast pain in premenopausal women. And from what we have heard, this seems to be amenable to treatment by placebo or acupuncture, danazol or bromocriptine, tamoxifen or various local agents which can be rubbed into the breast. Any of these treatment modalities seem to give some degree of response. I was interested particularly in the Hjørring experience where after treatment the patients relapsed at the rate of 50 per cent. In other words, some 50 per cent of the women stayed in remission. Perhaps it was a natural remission. Before I put too much emphasis on what I've learned about the therapy of this condition, I would like to know a great deal more about the natural history of breast pain in premenopausal women.

### Hughes

We have recently done a study of the natural history in patients who were studied first between 1972 and 1975 and followed up to 1977 and 1979, a period of about five years or so. In general, the natural history of severe disease (and this is what we are talking about, not the mild ones who respond to placebo) extends over a period of between 10 and 40 years. The earlier it occurs the longer it goes on for. It is certainly helped by some hormone-related conditions, the pill occasionally, pregnancy sometimes, the menopause finally. Patients who get severe mastalgia before the age of 20 are in for a very bad time.

I don't think it in the least surprising that there are relapses; it would be surprising if there were not. All we are doing is suppressing this natural process, producing an exaggeration of the normal cyclical changes within both the epithelium and the stroma of the lobule, both of which are hormone dependent, and I think we are seeing what one would expect. But if one treats patients with severe

*Benign Breast Disease, Edited by M. Baum, W. D. George, and L. E. Hughes, 1985: Royal Society of Medicine International Congress and Symposia series No. 76, published by the Royal Society of Medicine.*

mastalgia, one has no doubt that certain treatments are much more effective than others.

But as far as natural history is concerned, cyclical breast disease is a long-standing condition in severe cases, particularly when it starts early in reproductive life.

**George**

Just for our information, pre-publication, did you find out if there is any way you can decide on management on first presentation at the clinic? In other words, can you differentiate between groups who require different forms of treatment? Most people have the experience that the vast majority of patients who present with cyclical symptoms do not require very much in the way of active treatment. Do you have a technique whereby you can pick out the ones who should be started on an active agent on their first visit, as opposed to waiting to see?

**Hughes**

Well, first of all the patients are seen in a general breast clinic, so most of them never get to a mastalgia clinic. They are reassured and off they go and any pain they get is accepted as normal. They are then given breast-pain charts which they complete for three months. If it's found that their symptoms are very severe and their breast-pain charts show that their pain is both severe and prolonged, we would then consider treating them. So to some extent it's patient self-selection based on how severe the pain is. Only a very small proportion of the patient population needs treatment because pain for seven days before a period is totally normal. And pain—severe pain—for three weeks of the cycle is abnormal, with a continuum in between.

**George**

Any comment from Mr Mansel?

**Mansel**

Yes. I have in fact analysed the number of patients we treat as a proportion of the new patient case-load in the Cardiff breast clinic and it's only 4 per cent. People get the idea that we treat everybody and this is obviously not so. And this explains the fact that when one tries to run a trial on the condition, it's quite hard to find sufficient numbers of patients of the right type—those with severe pain. In the danazol trial I showed you, we ended up with a final number of 21 patients of the severe type with a mean duration of four years. Like everyone else, we reassure and send away most patients.

On another issue, I would like to answer the point raised by Mr Benson, rather provocatively. It is absolutely untrue that all agents work. All agents work only in open studies—that is the placebo effect. Yes, diuretics work—that too is a placebo effect. Progestogens have been looked at in double-blind studies of the premenstrual tension syndrome and have failed miserably against placebo, but it hasn't been done in breast disease. It certainly needs to be done, but it has to be done adequately.

**Preece**

Might I add a small point to that question of controlled studies? Usually we think that in setting up a placebo-controlled trial we are trying to establish that the agent that we think may be effective, really is effective. But it was most interesting to hear from Professor Goebel yesterday that, in a study that was not placebo-controlled, he failed to demonstrate the level of significant improvement that danazol showed amongst the group of treatments and hence gave, if I might suggest to Mr Benson, the impression that you indicated when you gave your question.

**Lloyd-Williams**

May I too take issue, slightly, with Mr Benson? In my experience it isn't so much the painful breasts—I think I now know what to do for patients who complain of pain in the breast. The patients who present a problem for me are those with a lump in the breast which is obviously hormonal. This is a problem for the surgeon but also for the patient who is very, very worried. This is very much a problem of hormonic modularity in the breast. The painful breast is by no means such a problem because, as has been adequately demonstrated here, there is a very good way of treating it.

**Benson**

I was adopting the role of *agent provocateur* and I seem to have succeeded in that role!

**George**

So do we all agree that this entity exists, although it's a relatively uncommon one? Or does anyone wish to cling to the theory that this might just be a variant of normality?

**Preece**

May I comment on the question of 'normality'? A study conducted at St Andrew's University some 10 or 20 years ago showed that of the young undergraduates there, the girls in their late 'teens and early twenties, 70 per cent experienced some premenstrual breast pain, and some were also aware that their breasts were lumpy. With regard to this question of nomenclature, it seems to me that we as clinicians have to approach epidemiologists to find out just what is the incidence of these symptoms in large populations in the areas in which we work. Surely statistics exist in epidemiological circles which would tell us what the incidence is of any particular anthropological feature which would make it normal? My suspicion is that we would find that a lot of this is indeed normal and this would help us, not only with the clinical components but also with the histopathological.

If I may further address this question of nomenclature, I would like to congratulate Dr Rasmussen again on the project he is involved with in Denmark. I think the serious attempt to do a scientific study over a long period has contributed greatly to our knowledge. I would, however, say to Dr Rasmussen, that I believe we have to resist the temptation to use histopathological, morphological terms for clinical and radiological entities. With regard to this word 'adenosis' for what to me looks just like diffuse radiodensity of the breast, I'd rather like that word—radiodensity—to be used, or even the Danish word for radiodensity, as long as that's all it meant.

**George**

Yes. The other problem with nomenclature is that it's very difficult to get pathologists to agree, not just the clinicians, the pathologists and the radiologists as well. On the question of the epidemiological distribution of breast symptoms within a population, has Mr Walsh got any information on the Liverpool screening programme?

**Walsh**

We have not yet analysed the data sufficiently. But there were nearly 300 women who provided luteal phase blood samples. These were well-women volunteers, presenting themselves for breast screening, so that this was a somewhat selected group, but about a quarter of their number admitted to persistent and severe to moderate cyclical breast discomfort of at least a week in nearly every cycle. Although the group was a selected one, it does indicate that a significant proportion of the population, possibly 20 or 25 per cent of premenopausal women between 30 and 50 years, are experiencing symptoms almost severe enough for them to seek medical attention.

**Mansel**

Recently published in the *American Journal of Epidemiology* was a study from Vancouver by Hislop in which nurses entering nursing school at about the age of 20 were looked at, and there was a 25- to 30-year follow-up. Breast size was documented on entry, breast symptoms, menstrual symptoms and many other variables of value in the epidemiology of breast disease. And on the basis of subsequent breast biopsy—which I think we'd all agree is a very good end-point—it was identified that there were characteristics even at the age of 20 in women who eventually had biopsy. One of these was menstrual irregularity, another was breast size—they had smaller breasts—and denser breasts, even when they were young. That's the only paper I know of that has addressed the question of epidemiology specifically, without looking specifically for breast cancer. The other point of interest, incidentally, was that the benign disease variables did not move in the same way as those for breast cancer risk factors, which is fascinating if we want to make the case that benign disease has nothing to do with breast cancer. This is certainly a useful contribution, but there is certainly a lack of good studies on the subject.

**George**

I think most people would agree that the entity exists, although it is not particularly common in its severe form. I think the results of the endocrine studies are interesting because it seems that this is a disease that is related to endocrine changes, inasmuch as it occurs at different points of the cycle, and yet no one has convincingly demonstrated any particular abnormality that is consistent amongst all groups. Would anyone care to comment on the endocrine results presented at this meeting, in particular on SHBG data presented this morning?

**Walsh**

I don't wish to detract from the undoubted benefits that can be achieved clinically with danazol, but I do think it's important to know what effects the endocrine manipulation we carry out are having on endogenous hormones, and possibly, as a consequence, the effects on histological appearances, because I think we have to remember, when treating these patients, that the spectre of breast cancer remains. Other drug treatments, such as the contraceptive pill, have rightly been scrutinized very closely for their effects. It's important to remember that the clinical presentation does not bear any relationship to the histological appearance and that certain proliferative histological appearances have been shown clearly to carry an increased risk of breast cancer. So clinical response may delude the clinician into thinking that all is well with his patient, not only symptomatically but also from the breast cancer risk point of view, when all the time the endogenous hormone balance may have been dangerously altered. I'm not suggesting this is happening, but I do think that we need to know more about this before many more women are treated for long periods, particularly patients whose biopsies may have demonstrated severe atypia of a degree which may put them in a high risk group. I think it is important, if we are going to embark on large-scale treatment for women at high risk, for us to know just what we are doing to their hormones.

**George**

That point is well taken.

**Perry**

The sex hormone-binding globulin (SHBG) falls in thyroid disease. I would like to ask the Danish group if they looked at concomitant thyroid function in any of their studies?

**Rasmussen**

We analysed TSH and we, of course, analysed T3, the best indicator of hyperthyroidism. We found no patients with higher levels. We did find two patients with hypothyroidism.

**George**

Would Dr Potts care to comment on some of the points raised by Mr Walsh, in relationship to exactly what danazol is doing to endogenous hormone levels? Particularly, perhaps, in relationship to dose, because quite a few speakers have brought up the question of the dose of the agent that should be used? It would certainly appear from the presentations this morning that 200 mg is as good as 400 mg, an experience shared by other groups. There is some suggestion that 100 mg was not all that different from 200 mg in the Scandinavian study. Other speakers have said that 50 mg once every other day is quite a good dose schedule. Dr Potts?

**Potts**

Perhaps I should speak on the effect of danazol on the normal hormonal pattern. If we go back to the early studies on endometriosis as well as fibrocystic breast disease, the total clinical picture indicates very strikingly that at the higher dosage levels, particularly

400 mg, 600 mg and 800 mg, we are affecting the FSH and LH surge during the ovulation phase to the degree that the oestrogen–progestin levels are affected, not to the base-line or minimal levels, but to the low–normal range over the entire cycle. So the hormonal pattern is one of a moderation in terms of oestrogen–progestin throughout the cycle. If we treat for, say, six months at the higher dosage levels, there will be anovulatory cycles, tendency for amenorrhoea, the oestrogen–progestin tending to be in the low–normal range. So we pretty much know what the steroid pattern is, what the gonadotropin pattern is.

In terms of the dosage, amongst our fibrocystic breast studies is a large multicentre study involving some 15 different investigators in 15 different sites, the data from which showed that the effect of danazol over the dosage range 100 mg, 200 mg, 400 mg, 600 mg, in terms of relief of pain and tenderness in particular, was rather strikingly non-dose-related. So it is not surprising that we are seeing effects, in the studies reported here, at lower dosage levels, particularly in terms of relief of pain and tenderness. If one considers a dosage of 100 mg, one sees that the effect on ovulation, the tendency to produce amenorrhoea, the effect on the steroidal pattern, are less apparent than they are at the 200–800 mg dosage levels. This brings into consideration a mechanism of action involving the competition with oestrogen–progestin, androgen receptors.

What we have concluded and are now recommending is that the starting dosage should be around 200 mg depending on the presenting symptoms, and increased or decreased according to the patient's response. Patients may well be maintained on a lower dose than the 200 mg starting dose, although they might need more. I mentioned the relief of pain and tenderness from a dosage standpoint; in our studies it became clear that these symptoms are markedly well relieved by danazol, the patient returning in four to six weeks much relieved, and after about eight weeks free from pain and tenderness. It will, however, take three to six months for the patient to be relieved of nodularity, or even longer, although there might be partial improvement in a shorter period of time. The follow-up recurrence rate seems to be related to the diminution of the nodularity, so that if you treat the patient for a six-month period or until the nodularity is controlled, the recurrence rate will be less and the duration of patient benefit will be longer.

### Morrison

I have enjoyed this symposium very much, but what I have found particularly stimulating is the way that scientific measurement is being brought to bear in relation to benign breast disease, something which is perhaps overdue. I am now keen to get back to Birmingham to organize my own data on this basis. But what has concerned me a little bit, particularly with regard to the placebo-controlled prospective randomized trials we have had presented, is the comparability of sequential measurements in individual patients. The importance of having one examiner has been emphasized; but we are dealing with a disease that is known to vary quite considerably throughout the menstrual cycle, and I don't believe that in any of the studies sufficient care has been taken to be absolutely sure that the measurements have been carried out at exactly the same point in the cycle, even perhaps as far as taking measurements at the same time of the day, in view of the data that have been presented about the swinging variation of hormonal levels during an individual's day. I would be interested to hear from those involved in such trials on this point.

**Doberl**

The point is well taken. However, even if one attempts to assess the patient at the same time in the cycle, that is, when the symptoms are at their worst, the picture becomes very quickly confused once the patient is on danazol, because, as you saw, even the lower dosage had a very considerable effect on the menstrual pattern, starting with irregularity and often proceeding to amenorrhoea. So once you have started danazol treatment, it is very hard to know exactly where in the menstrual cycle you are.

**Morrison**

What about the controls?

**Doberl**

There, of course, you can stick to regular intervals.

**George**

I quite agree, it is difficult. We certainly found that it is not easy to get multiple blood samples from women in the luteal phase, and the one thing that may solve the problem to some extent is the use of salivary steroid measurements, measuring free hormones, which might be more important anyway. This technique is not exactly widespread, but it is becoming slightly more available.

**Lloyd-Williams**

I find this all rather nebulous, this matter of measurement. It seems to me that whether it's a weighty breast or a heavy breast can be determined by measurement. Just as one can use thermography to measure changes in vascular pattern, one can devise methods to measure changes in the size of the breast, because there is no doubt that breast size does alter and in a cyclical way. Breast size can be measured by volume displacement, and the weight of the breast can be assessed by attaching a device to the straps of the bra', so that you can measure the effort needed to pull the breast up. Whilst the patient can tell you if their breasts feel heavy, what you are really trying to find out is how big they are and how dense they are, and so you need a method which combines both volume and weight in some way. So I think we should be looking at things like the vascular supply of the breast, at how it varies with the period (we can do this with scanning Doppler; we can do this with thermography), at the size of the breast and at the density of the breast.

One final thing, on the nodularity of the breast, I think people are inclined to forget that this is extraordinarily common. In the 12 000 screening series in Bath, 20 per cent of the women had what was described as nodular breasts. I think this is much more of a problem than the painful breast.

**George**

Well you have certainly thrown down a challenge to those of us with engineering interests!

**Watts**

I'm always intrigued by this question of heavy breasts and heavy tissue. It reminds me of Hamilton Bailey's heavy testes. Now the specific gravity of all soft tissue is almost identical. I've had patients who have tried to apply Archimedes' Principle to work out the size of their breasts, but neither they nor we have found the data derived of any value. I feel that we are dealing with matters which on the part of both patient and examiner are entirely subjective. Whether or not these things are common depends on how sympathetic is the surgeon; if he is sympathetic, he sees more patients with severe pain, more patients with very heavy breasts.

**George**

Whilst accepting what you say, I feel we still have to try to go for some form of objective measurement, if at all possible. Certainly, when we looked at mammographic pattern against nodularity we found that they do not seem to correlate at all. So it's very difficult to know what you are dealing with sometimes.

**Lloyd-Williams**

On the subject of low doses of danazol, although I don't have statistical proof or numbers, it seems to me that it's a good idea to titrate the dose of danazol against the patient's pain. It so happens that I have a patient who has herself titrated the dose down to 25 mg. If you think of what's involved in breaking up a danazol capsule to get a dose of 25 mg, you will see that it requires a great deal of ingenuity on the patient's part. But I have an intelligent patient who has done this and takes the dose for six days before her period. I know that one swallow doesn't make a summer, but we are talking about subjective things, and if a patient is better on low dosage, as far as I'm concerned, that's fine. I did wonder if there was any scientific proof for a low-dose effect, and I think there is some scientific evidence that danazol has a local effect on the receptors.

**George**

Before we conclude, I think we should discuss the place of different agents in the treatment of painful breast disease or nodular breast disease. What do people think generally?

**Hinton**

I think the thing which has emerged most from the Nottingham breast pain clinic is the small numbers of patients who actually need treatment of any kind. We have had some 300 patients at the breast pain clinic for treatment out of something like 2000 seen in the general clinic complaining of breast pain over the years that we have been running the clinics. There is a large group of these patients in whom almost any agent will work; about 40 or 50 per cent seem to respond to anything. But, certainly, since we've been using danazol the response rate has gone up to 80 or 90 per cent. The patients who are very difficult, and the ones for whom I would appreciate advice, are the ones who do not respond to danazol, because at the present time I do not know how to manage these patients at all, and these are the patients who come demanding subcutaneous mastectomy and occasionally persuade me to do so.

**Mansel**

I don't think we should give every patient danazol. As we've said, the selection of patients is important. What I'd like to see is the adequate assessment of agents which have not been properly tested. As I've mentioned before, progestogen needs to be assessed carefully, especially in view of the epidemiology from the Oxford unit and others, showing that if progestogens are taken for a long time, patients get less benign breast disease. There are, of course, other agents that need looking at; from America there is news of caffeine; some people are looking at prostaglandins. Really, we've got to understand what is going on and that is the way forward. We have to know what is going on in the breast-cell, and that might have a spin-off also for the understanding of cancer.

**Fossard**

I would like to take Mr Mansel's argument a little bit further. It has been mentioned only briefly at this symposium that the breast is a target organ and I can't help feeling that some of the controversy that surrounds the different treatments that have been used arises from the failure of all of us to understand what happens to the breast in response to the treatment that is given, or the indirect effects of that treatment upon the endogenous hormones. It's not the fact that levels change within the plasma but the consequences of these changes upon the breast itself that influence whether or not a patient gets a good response to a treatment or a poor response. It does not seem to me that this aspect has been examined at all. But I'm no expert on this condition: I'm here to learn.

**George**

I take your point. I think that end-organ sensitivity is an important factor but it is a very, very difficult thing to measure, and this is part of the problem.

**Gorins**

The problem of the choice of dosage of danazol is not a difficult one; it depends on whether or not you wish to inhibit ovulation. On 400 mg daily you are sure to inhibit ovulation; inhibition of ovulation on 200 mg a day is uncertain. Someone mentioned a pregnancy on this dosage. With 100 mg daily there is no inhibition of ovulation but it is possible that there is an action on the target cells. I believe that danazol acts in two ways: first by blocking ovulation, by virtue of its antigonadotropin activity, and also by an atrophic effect on the target cells. If you use 400 mg a day you should warn your patients that they are likely to have disordered menstruation. It is important that they are informed of this possibility in advance and also of the possibility of weight gain. We always advise our patients to pursue a low calorie, low lipid diet whilst on danazol to avoid weight gain.

**Preece**

I have a few comments on Mr Hinton's question on the treatment of difficult, danazol-resistant cases. During this symposium, a number of people have spoken of such patients in their practice and Dr Rasmussen demonstrated beautifully the value of close documentation and study of one such case, which revealed a huge amount of information. I think we should not feel discouraged by patients of this kind but should continue to keep in touch with them and document the details of them carefully to see what happens to them. One very instructive lesson which was learned from one such case in Newcastle, which had come to subcutaneous mastectomy, was that there is much to be said for a very careful psychological assessment of these patients, not only by the simple indices, like the Crown-–Crisp Experimental Index of the Middlesex Hospital questionnaire, which can be given in five or 10 minutes and can give you a good idea as to whether the patient is neurotic, but also by collaboration with a psychiatrist or social worker. The Newcastle case demonstrated very well that although subcutaneous mastectomy was the right treatment for that patient, the patient was helped only by a combination of psychotherapy and surgery.

**George**

I think it is quite clear that we need still to continue to look at the endocrine profiles in these women and perhaps salivary assays will help. It appears to me that the question of dosage of danazol remains an open one. Listening to people who use the drug a lot gives me the impression that there is a tendency to use lower and lower doses. If that is really the case, then it seems that we should be looking not only at the endocrine effects of low dosages but also at the clinical effects of such dosages.

I get the impression also that the vast majority of women who present with breast symptoms do not require any particularly active treatment beyond reassurance and that it is only a minority that will require danazol. We still need to look not only at danazol critically but at other agents too, such as progestogens, as suggested by Mr Mansel.

I now bring this session to a close, with my thanks on your behalf to Sterling-Winthrop for organizing what has been a very enjoyable and most informative symposium.

I would like, too, to thank all the speakers and all those who participated in the discussions. Thank you all.

# Summing-up

THE RT. HON. THE LORD PORRITT, GCMG, GCVO, CBE

Ladies and gentlemen, I have the feeling that you share with me a certain amount of regret that this very happy and most useful symposium on benign breast disease is drawing to a close.

We have had summaries of the individual presentations, we have had summaries of each of the sessions and we have just had a summary of the whole symposium, and so there is little left for me to do. However, in view of the fact that as long ago as 30 years I was very actively engaged in dealing with this particular group of diseases, in which I had great interest, I hope you will allow me to give you a few of my impressions of the matters discussed at this meeting.

First and foremost, I am intrigued by how much has changed in the approach to this problem. I am equally intrigued by how much has not changed, and I think this is all to the good.

The symposium opened with the question of terminology, a subject which has occupied a good deal of the time during the last two days. I am going to refer to it yet again because I consider terminology to be a matter of very considerable importance. There is no doubt that the clinical and pathological terminology has become more and more involved and the problem therefore progressively more complicated. And because we do feel that this is an important group of diseases, there is an obvious need for terminology both simple and international. At the discussions here, we have been using a number of different terms to describe exactly the same thing, and we have been describing a whole lot of different things with exactly the same term. This is most confusing and possibly also dangerous. It is not easy to suggest a remedy but, as with so many other things in life, a return to simplicity would be a step in the right direction.

As has been said here often enough, this group of diseases manifests itself as pain, tension and tenderness, and nodularity, and my suggestion is that the terminology should concentrate on these three things that the patient complains of.

Passing on—as we did—to the laboratory investigation of benign breast disease, it is most stimulating to hear of the very definite advances that have been made in biochemistry, in cytology, in pharmacology, in radiology and in all the other scientific areas. There is no doubt that we are now much better informed, but are we very much wiser? We have not yet discovered the aetiology of these diseases, not by a long way, and I think Professor Baum summed up the position perfectly when he said, in effect, 'We don't know what to call them and we don't know what causes them, so let's get on with the treatment.' Certainly this was an appropriate thing to say but somewhat alarming also, because it means that we have been discussing an empirical problem.

But let me not depress you; the sessions that followed, on the pharmacology and

*Benign Breast Disease, Edited by M. Baum, W. D. George, and L. E. Hughes, 1985: Royal Society of Medicine International Congress and Symposia series No. 76, published by the Royal Society of Medicine.*

the clinical use of danazol, achieved an extraordinary consensus of opinion on this therapeutic agent. I listened with great interest to the series of very well-carried-out and in many ways quite different investigations that have been conducted in the UK and in various other parts of Europe—in Germany, in France and in Scandinavia. All reached the same conclusion—that in danazol we have a drug almost before its time.

I was particularly impressed by the Hjørring project, a magnificent experiment, beautifully organized and extremely well carried out. And it continues, I am glad to say.

Which leads me to conclude that we have decided that this group of diseases has a hormonal origin, an endocrinological origin; we can at least say that. We are able also to say that this is a group of diseases for which we have found, empirically, a potent, safe, although sadly rather expensive, therapeutic agent.

As a somewhat ancient chairman, I propose to take the privilege of mentioning three more matters discussed at this conference and which struck me as particularly interesting.

The first was the idea produced by Mr Kissin about the use of danazol in unmasking breast carcinoma. It would, of course, extend the field significantly if this technique proved to be really worthwhile and really safe. Because, if we are honest, the importance of this conference, and it has hardly been mentioned, is really related to cancer of the breast. This group of diseases, which we call benign breast disease, is important mostly because of its relationship to cancer.

The patients who come to you are in the main concerned about whether or not they have cancer. Of course they have pain and they have discomfort, but they also have fear. That is my first point.

My second concerns the use of mammography at relatively frequent and short intervals. I am very sorry but I find that hard to justify as a method of assessing results. The devices used may be very well controlled and protected but their use in this way worries me.

Lastly, I mention the point made by Professor Gorins regarding the psychological condition of the patient, an aspect of benign breast disease to which, in my view, insufficient attention is paid. Anyone who is a good doctor is, or should be, a good psychologist also. Cancer phobia is a very dire and definite condition and its possibility must be kept in mind when treating the patient with benign breast disease. Let us remember that the breast is not only a potential milk-factory, it is also a very obvious sex-characteristic and of vast personal importance to its owner. It behoves us to bear that in mind and not to treat the breast in isolation, as it were, from the patient who owns it.

This has been a very well-argued symposium. I have enjoyed it and I get the feeling that all of you have too. I hope it will lead to further developments, an increase in knowledge and even in wisdom! Then it will lead to advances at a rate sufficiently fast to warrant another symposium on danazol whilst I am still alive!

My final duty is to express on behalf of us all our very genuine thanks, first of all to our three chairmen of sessions who, I suggest, have been exceptionally good; they have led and directed and controlled their sessions with the greatest of tact and success. Secondly, I express our thanks to the excellent speakers, particularly the Continental speakers who have coped with the language difficulties so well, for the splendid papers they have all produced and presented so effectively.

My thanks to you, too, for being such an intelligent, interested and responsive audience, for the way you have participated and taken part in the discussions.

Not least, thanks are due to Sterling-Winthrop for their magnificent organization of this symposium and for the efficient way in which we have been looked after.

# A useful clinical classification of benign breast disease
H. JUNKERMANN *et al.*

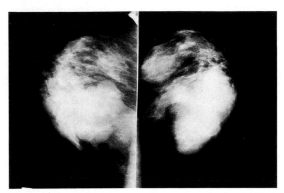

Fig. 1. Mammogram of gross cystic disease, showing opacities with a clearly defined margin.

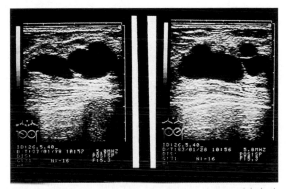

Fig. 2. Ultrasonograph visualization of multiple large cysts.

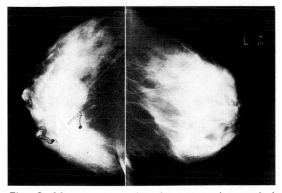

Fig. 3. Mammogram showing several rounded structures in left breast. Sonography demonstrated a cyst at (1) and a tumour at (2). (See Fig. 4.)

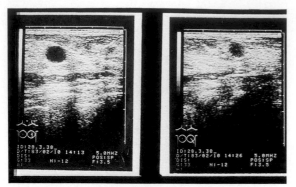

*Fig. 4. Ultrasonograph visualization of a cyst, with no echoes from within, and a fibroadenoma. Same patient as in Fig. 3.*

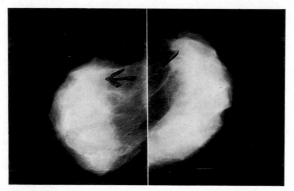

*Fig. 5. Mammogram of patient diagnosed radiologically and clinically as a case of benign breast disease.*

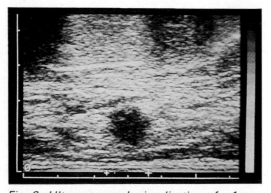

*Fig. 6. Ultrasonograph visualization of a 1 cm carcinoma. Same patient as in Fig. 5.*

# The contribution of infra-red thermography to the diagnosis of benign breast disease A. GORINS *et al.*

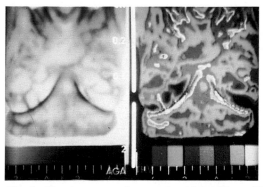

*Fig. 1. Thermogram of normal subject (Type C). A diversified venous network is shown.*

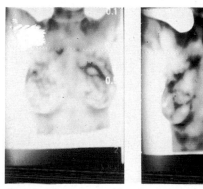

*Fig. 2. Thermographic changes which occur in the course of the menstrual cycle. Left: beginning of cycle; right: end of cycle, showing clear increase in vascularization. It is this phenomenon which leads to the recommendation that thermography be carried out at the beginning of the menstrual cycle.*

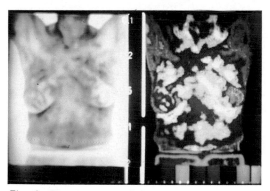

*Fig. 3. Thermogram of a peri-menopausal woman, showing very high temperature and considerable vascularization.*

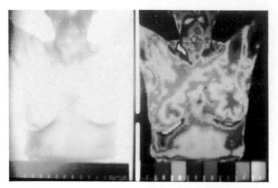

*Fig. 4. Same patient as in Fig. 3: confirmed menopause.*

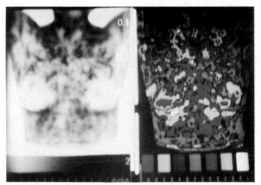

*Fig. 5. Thermogram of a woman suffering from neuro-vegetative dystonia, illustrating the so-called 'L' (for leopard-like) pattern.*

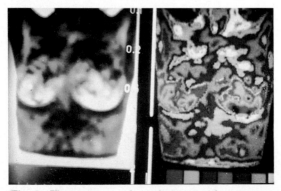

*Fig. 6. Thermogram of another case of neuro-vegetative dystonia.*

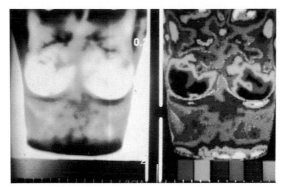

Fig. 7. Same patient as in Fig. 6, after a walk lasting 1·5 h, showing significant cooling.

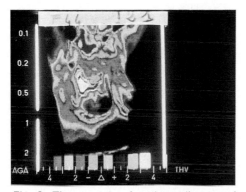

Fig. 8. Thermogram showing a 'hot spot' of more than 3 °C, indicative of cancer.

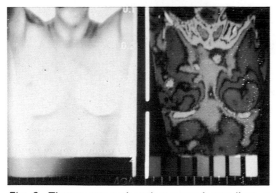

Fig. 9. Thermogram showing a moderate 'hot spot' of 2 °C, indicative of a benign lesion.

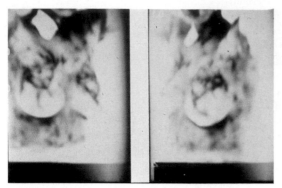

Fig. 10. Thermogram of patient with benign dystrophy (three-quarter and front views). The rich vascular network is clearly seen.

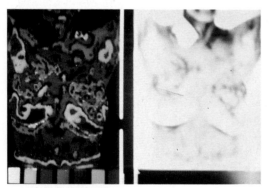

Fig. 11. Thermogram demonstrating breast dystrophy, showing thick vascularization with peri-mammillary ring.

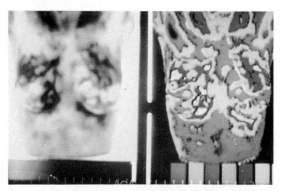

Fig. 12. Thermogram of patient with hypermastia and dystrophy.

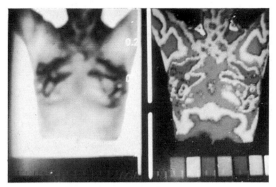

*Fig. 13. Thermogram showing a 'fir-tree' arrangement of vessels.*

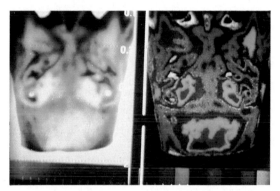

*Fig. 14. Thermogram showing breast dystrophy and peri-mammillary ring.*

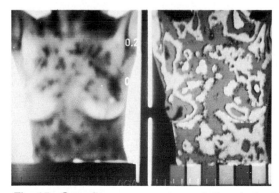

*Fig. 15. Complex case: neuro-vegetative dystonia with appearance of dystonia and cancer 'hot spot' (left breast).*

# Comparison of danazol with taxoxifen, gestagen, acupuncture, local treatment and placebo: results in one thousand patients

W. EGGERT-KRUSE *et al.*

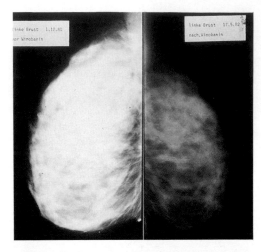

*Fig. 1. Left: mammogram showing severe dense fibrocystic disease. Right: same patient after six months' treatment with danazol 200 mg daily. Note reduction in breast size and density and improved radiographic transparency.*

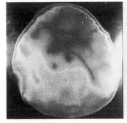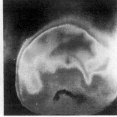

*Fig. 2. Left: thermogram showing massive hyperthermia with an irregular vascular pattern. Right: after six months' danazol 200 mg daily, thermogram shows considerable reduction in breast temperature and normalization of vascular pattern.*

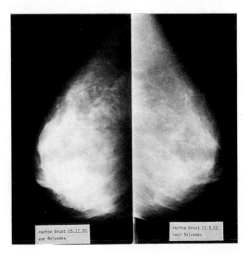

*Fig. 3. Left: pre-treatment mammogram. Right: after six months' treatment with 100 mg tamoxifen daily. Note marked reduction in tissue density.*

# Experience with danazol in the UCH Breast Clinic: an open study
N. B. SHAIKH

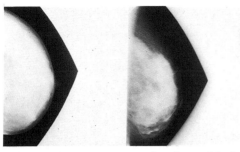

*Fig. 5. Left: mammogram of patient with six-month history of severe breast pain, showing large areas of density (nodular patchiness) in supra-areolar regions. Right: mammogram of same patient after three months' danazol treatment.*

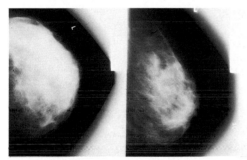

*Fig. 6. Left: pre-danazol mammogram of post-hysterectomy patient. Right: mammogram of same patient after six-months' danazol treatment, showing reduction in nodularity.*

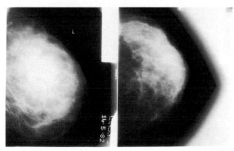

*Fig. 7. Left: pre-danazol mammogram showing firm mass. Right: post-danazol, the breast had become smaller and the mass had disappeared.*

# Double-blind crossover study of danazol versus placebo in the treatment of severe fibrocystic breast disease A. GORINS et al.

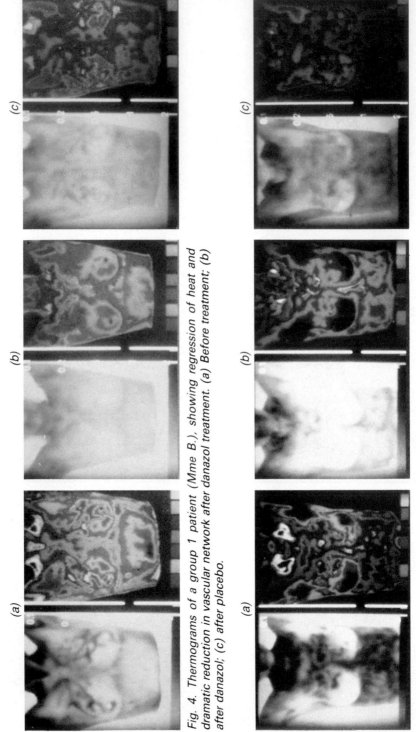

Fig. 4. Thermograms of a group 1 patient (Mme B.), showing regression of heat and dramatic reduction in vascular network after danazol treatment. (a) Before treatment; (b) after danazol; (c) after placebo.

Fig. 5. Thermograms of a group 1 patient (Mme C.), showing regression of heat and dramatic reduction in vascular network after danazol treatment. (a)–(c) as in Fig. 4.

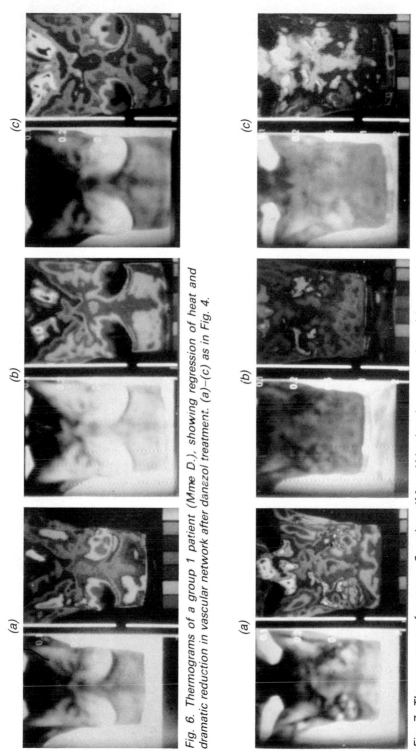

*Fig. 6. Thermograms of a group 1 patient (Mme D.), showing regression of heat and dramatic reduction in vascular network after danazol treatment. (a)–(c) as in Fig. 4.*

*Fig. 7. Thermograms of a group 2 patient (Mme H.), showing regression of heat and dramatic reduction in vascular network after danazol treatment. (a) Before treatment; (b) after placebo; (c) after danazol.*

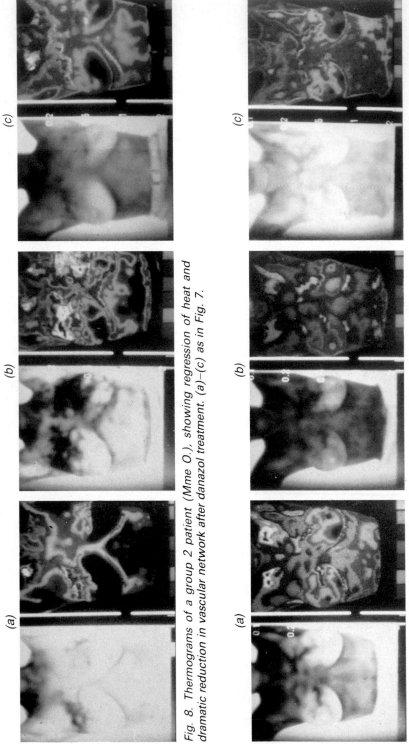

*Fig. 8. Thermograms of a group 2 patient (Mme O.), showing regression of heat and dramatic reduction in vascular network after danazol treatment. (a)–(c) as in Fig. 7.*

*Fig. 9. Thermograms of a group 2 patient (Mme P.), showing regression of heat and dramatic reduction in vascular network after danazol treatment. (a)–(c) as in Fig. 7.*